In Good Health

GESCHICHTE UND
PHILOSOPHIE
DER MEDIZIN

HISTORY AND
PHILOSOPHY
OF MEDICINE

Herausgegeben von
Andreas Frewer

Band 9

Almut Caspary

In Good Health

Philosophical-Theological Analysis
of the Concept of Health
in Contemporary Medical Ethics

Franz Steiner Verlag Stuttgart 2010

*Gedruckt mit Hilfe der Geschwister Boehringer
Ingelheim Stiftung für Geisteswissenschaften
in Ingelheim am Rhein*

Umschlagabbildungen:
1. Die Ärzte Hippokrates und Galen (links) im
   Fachdisput. Fresko (13. Jh.) in der Krypta der
   Kirche von Anagni, Latium (Italien).
2. Human embryonic stem cell.
   © Wellcome Images

Reihenherausgeber:
Professor Dr. Andreas Frewer, M.A.
Institut für Geschichte und Ethik der Medizin
Universität Erlangen-Nürnberg
Glückstr. 10
91054 Erlangen

Bibliografische Information der Deutschen
Nationalbibliothek:
Die Deutsche Nationalbibliothek verzeichnet diese
Publikation in der Deutschen Nationalbibliografie;
detaillierte bibliografische Daten sind im Internet über
<http://dnb.d-nb.de> abrufbar.

ISBN 978-3-515-09318-7

ACKNOWLEDGEMENTS

I am indebted to the many people and institutions who accompanied and supported me on the journey of reading and writing that led to this book.

My first words of thanks must go to Dr. Michael Banner, now Trinity College Cambridge. He supervised my work having introduced me to Augustine when I came to King's College London in 1999. A rigorous and analytical thinker as well as one of the most musical writers I know, he never failed to open up new dimensions, provoke further thoughts, and encourage me to carry on.

I am grateful to Prof. Peter Byrne, King's College London, as well as to the Systematic Theology Postgraduate Seminar and the Interdisciplinary Postgraduate Seminar on Law and Theology in Medical Ethics, both Humboldt-University Berlin, for discussing ideas and sharing concerns. Throughout, Moira Langston has provided all possible administrative support and helped patiently with all formalities involved.

This book would not have been possible without sources of financial and institutional support: resources were made available by the Franz-Steiner-Verlag, the Wellcome Images for the cover photograph, and last but not least the Geschwister-Boehringer-Ingelheim-Stiftung with a generous grant for printing costs. My special thanks goes to Prof. Andreas Frewer, University Erlangen-Nuremberg and editor of the series "History and Philosophy of Medicine", a most assiduous supervisor of the editing process.

I could not have undertaken this journey without the continuous love and support of my family and friends in Germany, the United Kingdom and elsewhere. They all helped in their many inimitable ways. Above all, I am deeply grateful to my parents, my sisters and my grandmother. My additional thanks goes to those who read drafts of this work, in particular Joy Howard, Dr. Marius Chan and Dr. Rod Taylor.

Finally, thank you Leah and George for your patience and conviviality – from London to Berlin to Edinburgh and back to Berlin. I wonder where our journey will take us next.

Almut Caspary
Berlin-Friedenau
Summer 2010

CONTENTS

1. INTRODUCTION

Medical research inspires hope. It promises novel therapies, a decrease of pain and suffering, and an increase of health. Numbers of patients and their families await cures for devastating diseases. They are hopeful of medicine's ability to provide relief from much human misery. Many of us, perhaps even most of us, welcome medical research, new medical technologies, and therapeutic advances. Modern medicine excites admiration. At the same time, we hear the warning voices of those who anticipate dangers and risks of certain technologies both for individuals and societies, and of those who fear that some medical projects might tempt us to transcend the limits of our bodily existence.

With a similar mixture of welcoming excitement, hopeful anticipation, and cautioning concern German parliamentarians discussed embryonic stem cell research in late January 2002. The German Bundestag frequently referred to the United Kingdom as example of responsible promotion of research. While the legislative outcome was to differ significantly,[1] the debate itself showed no substantial difference to that in the United Kingdom: advocates of embryonic stem cell research referred to its therapeutic potential, the possibilities of health for the individual or groups of individuals, and to society's moral obligation of healing.[2] Yet, what some heralded as a breakthrough for health or cause for hope, others – and amongst those also patient support groups – rejected for fear of discrimination. Would money not be spent more sensibly on support structures for the disabled here and now, rather than on research of unclear therapeutic potential?[3]

---

1   The production of stem cell lines is prohibited in Germany. However, stem cells can be imported as long as they are derived from lines created outside Germany and prior to a specified date. In the 2002 debate, the cut-off date was fixed as 31st January 2002. In April 2008, the German Bundestag moved the cut-off date to 1st May 2007. "The result can be interpreted as a confirmation of the compromise made in 2002: the general ban on creating and working on human embryonic stem cell lines in Germany is upheld; however, it will still be possible to import cell lines that were harvested abroad prior to a cut-off date." (http://www.eurostemcell.org/commentanalysis/german-parliament-passes-amendment-stem-cell-act, last accessed 01/2010).

2   See the references made to an "ethics of healing" in the contributions of (mainly Christian Democrat) MPs who supported either the use of embryos for embryonic stem cell research in Germany or at least the import of stem cell lines created prior to 31.01.2002: e.g. Peter Hintze (CDU), Ulrike Flash (FDP), Katherina Reiche (CDU), Maria Böhmer (CDU). Those who were more sceptical regarding the use of embryos for research criticised arguments of health benefits: e.g. Andrea Fischer (SPD), Monika Griefahn (SPD), Ernst Ulrich von Weizsäcker (SPD), Christa Nickels (Green), Ilja Seifert (PDS), Hubert Hüppe (CDU), Hermann Kues (CDU). Cf. transcript of the 214. German parliamentary debate, 30.01.2002, http://dip21.bundestag.de/dip21/btp/14/212/14214212.00.pdf, last accessed 01/2010.

3   Cf. Ilja Seifert, http://dip21.bundestag.de/dip21/btp/14/212/14214212.00.pdf, last accessed 01/2010.

Listening to the 2002 debate and thinking over these concerns, questions arose that largely covered the following two areas: (1) What *is* human life that is to be cured and cared for? Are our assessments of medical research based on a certain vision of human life, and if so, what vision is this? What understanding of the *body* (the biological aspects of human life), and of human *personhood* (that which makes human life particular, unique, *my* life or *your* life) is the foundation of moral arguments in medicine? (2) What is health? How is health understood where it is used as an argument in favour of, for instance, embryonic stem cell research? Where value is attributed to health, even to the *potential* of health, what underscores the moral claim of cure and relief of suffering?

Do we know the answers to these questions? Or do we possess, and refer to, a set of incoherent, fragmented survivals from moral knowledge and tradition, as Alasdair MacIntyre famously suggests in *After Virtue*[4] when he says,

> "Ill-assorted conceptual fragments from various parts of our past are deployed together in private and public debates which are notable chiefly for the unsettable character of the controversies thus carried on and the apparent arbitrariness of each of the contending parties."[5]

This suspicion of MacIntyre's prompted me in 2002 to explore further the above questions, and in doing so, the nature of moral knowledge and tradition in the area of medicine, medical research and health care. MacIntyre's suspicion of "ill-assorted conceptual fragments" led to a desire to understand the object and end of medicine, and the anthropological assumptions that underlie the morality of medical research and clinical practice.[6] To this end, I turned to modern philosophical accounts of health in relation to pre-modern philosophies of medicine and theological (Christian) anthropology.

In the Christian tradition, excellent work has been done on health and medicine.[7] The present study will fall short of volumes such as Stanley S. Harakas'

---

4   MacIntyre (1985), *After Virtue*.
5   Ibid., 256.
6   Note: By 'medical' and 'medicine' I mean *clinical medicine from the Western perspective*.
     I try to avoid terms such as 'scientific' medicine or 'biomedicine' as they carry the implication of a monolithic system beyond the reach and influence of culture. Social scientists have demonstrated significant variation in biomedical notions and clinical practices, see for instance, Hahn/Gaines (1985), *Physicians of Western Medicine: Anthropological Approaches to Theory and Practice*; Lock (1993), *Encounters with Aging: Mythologies of Menopause in Japan and North America*; Wright/Treacher (1982), *The Problem of Medical Knowledge: Examining the Social Construction of Medicine*. For the terminological distinction of biomedicine and holistic medicine see also Guttmacher (1979), "Whole in Body, Mind and Spirit: Holistic Health and the Limits of Medicine". I will not consider alternative Western medicines such as homeopathic medicine or Asian medicines often termed 'traditional' medicines.
7   Apart from the numerous articles that focus on one particular theologian, schools of theology or particular aspects of medicine, I have in mind here the excellent series *Health/Medicine in the Faith Traditions* with volumes on Health and Medicine in the Anglican, Catholic, Eastern Orthodox, Lutheran, Methodist, and Reformed Tradition as well as Hindu, Islamic and Jewish Tradition respectively (published by the Park Ridge Center for the Study of Health, Faith, and Ethics, Chicago).

Health and Medicine in the Eastern Orthodox Tradition[8] and Martin E. Marty's *Health and Medicine in the Lutheran Tradition.*[9] Yet unlike these two (and similar others), I do not aim to present one particular tradition of thought and its relationship to medical healing. I will look at Christian theology, its philosophical ancestry and present day philosopher companions[10] and will develop an account of health and healing which is largely based on an Augustinian anthropology (Augustine himself, though a saint only in the Catholic or Anglo-Catholic tradition, played and plays a prominent role in the development of Calvinist and Lutheran doctrines, too). I seek dialogue with representative voices of Orthodox theology past and present. Indeed, my aim is *to dialogue* with thinkers who were concerned with health throughout the ages – from the beginnings of rational medicine through to the present times. Half of the writers I engage with lived and wrote in the first millennium. They were either directly involved in the shaping of rational medicine as the art of curing *and* caring, or responded vividly – and at times sharply – to medicine's emerging doctrines. The other half, living and writing now or in the last century of the second millennium, was at the centre of health debates in the context of scientific medicine as we know it today.

Comparing and contrasting the interpretations of health of those who influenced medicine in its very beginnings, as well as of those who accompany its present activities, allows me to identify significant traits and/or interpretative gaps of the concept of health. Engaging with the writers of different traditions permits the explanation of how a *unitive* understanding of the natural body in its personal, social and cultural aspects may enable today's physicians to conceptualise their actions as reading natural given-ness in dialogue with their patients' personal views of disease and health in the context of social, political and cultural norms.

I will show how an orientation of human action towards God's love – which is crucial for Augustine's understanding of human morality and ethics – may direct both physicians and patients to the horizon of ultimate questions concerned with human striving for fulfilment in the face of the limitations imposed by death.

This, then, may sum up the contribution of this study to the field of medical morality and medical practice. With *critical* dialogue at its centre – a dialogue with a selection of theologians (both of East and West) and philosophers (both of past and present) – it develops an account of medicine's end that is original in its *proceedings*: it links historical and contemporary reflection on medicine, medical research and health care; it looks at the birth of modern medicine in order to understand its goals and practices today; it draws out historical and conceptual

---

8   Stanley S. Harakas, *Health and Medicine in the Eastern Orthodox Tradition* (Crossroad/New York, 2000).

9   Martin E. Marty, *Health and Medicine in the Lutheran Tradition* (Crossroad/New York, 1998).

10   In its philosophical aspects the present study might bear some resemblance with philosophical contributions such as Leon Kass' "The End of Medicine and the Pursuit of Health" (1975), and more recently Daniel Callahan/Eric Parens' "The Ends of Medicine: Shaping New Goals" (1995), as well as in German language Dirk Lanzerath's *Krankheit und ärztliches Handeln* (2000).

connections between the first millennium thinkers and contemporary theology and philosophy in order to identify characteristics of the concept of health; it takes seriously the relevance of the historical past as located in the present through the time-transcending spirit.

1.1 OVERVIEW OF KEY LITERATURE AND IDEAS

Health is the end of medicine. The 1964 *Declaration of Helsinki* states as a recommendation for physicians in biomedical research involving human subjects,

> "It is the mission of the physician to safeguard the health of the people. His or her knowledge and conscience are dedicated to the fulfilment of this mission."[11]

In most cultures explanatory concepts of health and disease have been developed. As Egyptian papyri and Mesopotamian medical texts show these concepts had far-reaching consequences for diagnosis and therapy, for healers' and patients' attitudes to each other and to their dealings with disease, for social reactions and care structures, and for the cultural significance of diseases.

Exploring dimensions and changes in the concepts of disease and health in the course of history and across past societies and cultures, medical historians have distinguished four causal categories: (1) Disease and health are attributed to the interplay between liquid and solid components of the body (e.g. Greek Hippocratic and Indian Ayurvedic medicine); (2) Disease and health are attributed to the relationship of body and spirit or the natural and the supernatural (found in most religious traditions); (3) Diseases are existing external entities such as demons, bacteria or viruses (ontological notion of disease); (4) Diseases are the consequence of disturbed biological functions within individuals (the so-called physiological notion of disease) and may result from either an individual's biological, psychological or spiritual disposition (endogenous) and/or external factors such as climate, food intake, supernatural powers or natural entities (exogenous).[12]

---

11   Declaration of Helsinki: http://bmj.bmjjournals.com/cgi/content/full/313/7070/1448/a, last accessed 01/2010. Cf. also Schmidt/Frewer (eds.), *History and Theory of Human Experimentation. The Declaration of Helsinki and Modern Medical Ethics* (2007).

12   The literature on the history of the concept of disease and health is ample. The following (chronological) list presents but a small selection on which the above summary drew; it includes some of the most influential monographs as well as overviews given in articles. Cf. Sigerist, *Civilisation and Disease* (1943); Berghoff, *Entwicklungsgeschichte des Krankheitsbegriffs* (1947); Risse, *The Conception of Disease* (1953); Temkin, *The Scientific Approach to Disease: Specific Entity and Individual Sickness* (1963); Edelstein, *Ancient Medicine* (1967); Schipperges/Seidler/Unschuld, *Krankheit, Heilkunst, Heilung* (1978); Temkin, *Health and Disease* (1973); Rothschuh, *Was ist Krankheit? Erscheinung, Erklärung, Sinndeutung* (1995); Risse, "Health and Disease–History of the Concepts" (1978); v. Engelhardt, *Health and Disease–History of the Concepts* (1995) as well as Schäfer/Frewer/Schockenhoff/Wetzstein, *Gesundheitskonzepte im Wandel* (2008).

With regard to the relevance of these categories for present day medicine, historian of medicine Owsei Temkin remarks,

> "Of the stages through which these ideas have gone, some belong to the past, others have merely seen a metamorphosis. Disease as a physiological process and disease as an entity are recurrent themes which have been likened to the struggle between nominalism and realism. [...] *The history of the ideas of health and disease cannot decide these issues; it can only present them.*"[13]

Health and disease are also (and have always been) themes in art,[14] philosophy,[15] religion,[16] and more recently in the social sciences, in particular medical anthropology,[17] psychology, sociology and social theory.[18] Such wide-ranging interest immediately points to the difficulties one faces when trying to explain the concepts in medical terms only: Health and disease are complex, ambiguous, and multidimensional terms.

---

13 Temkin, "Health and Disease", 406 (my italics).
14 In literature examples range from the Old Testament's book of Job to Leo Tolstoy's *The Death of Ivan Illich* to Thomas Mann's *Magic Mountain*. Disease in 19th and 20th century literature is also one of the themes in Susan Sontag's 1978 *Illness as Metaphor*.
15 Plato's, Aristotle's and Galen's ideas on health and medicine are at the centre of chapter three of this study. For further key texts, see the utopian writings of Thomas Moore (1478–1535) and Francis Bacon (1561–1626) which include guiding principles for eugenic health policies; Rene Descartes (1596–1650) mechanical model of health and disease bound up with his dualist anthropology; G. F. Hegel (1770–1831) *Philosophy of Nature,* which emphasises the victory of the spirit over disease and death. Eminent physicians-philosophers were Thomas Sydenham, G. B. Morgan, Xavier Bichat, Claude Bernard, and Rudolf Virchow. Aside from the substantial medical philosophy debate on health which is the focus of chapter five, the 20th century would not be complete without philosopher-physician Karl Jaspers "Die Begriffe Gesundheit und Krankheit" (1973), Michel Foucault's *The Birth of the Clinic: An Archaeology of Medical Perception* (1973), Georges Canguilhem's *On the Normal and the Pathological* (1978) and H. G. Gadamer's *Über die Verborgenheit der Gesundheit* (2003).
16 For an overview on world religions and health, see Tillich, "The Relation of Religion and Health: Historical Considerations and Theoretical Questions" (1946); Sullivan, *Healing and Restoring. Health and Medicine in the World's Religious Traditions* (1989).
17 Apart from 'classical' anthropological and ethnographic case studies, anthropologists are often also interested in the power relations that lead to one particular set of interpretations becoming the dominant and "authentic" set of meanings. Cf. also Young, "The Anthropologies of Illness and Sickness" (1982); Latour/Woolgar, *Laboratory Life: The Construction of Scientific Fact* (1986); Pfleiderer/Bichmann, *Krankheit und Kultur. Eine Einführung in die Ethnomedizin* (1985).
18 One tradition within the sociology of health and disease focuses on how the distribution of death and disease is influenced by factors such as age, gender, race, and social class. This tradition can be traced back to French sociologist Emile Durkheim's work on suicide (1890s). The second tradition is oriented to the physician-patient relationship and is interested in the meanings of disease for each of them, and how their interpretations reflect the power hierarchies in society. This tradition began in the 1950s with Talcott Parson's discussion of the sick role (*The Social System,* 1951) and has been taken up and developed by medical psychology in particular.

They have personal, cultural, and social dimensions. In the words of medical historian Dietrich von Engelhardt,

> "Sickness and health in their natural and cultural breadth, remind medicine of its fundamentally scientific and humanistic nature. Health and disease are concerned with life and death, and are closely connected to the physical, social, psychic, and spiritual nature of humans."[19]

Whilst historians of medicine reflect on health and disease in their different cultural and societal contexts in the light of historical sources, thus uncovering the roots of modern day approaches, the philosophy of medicine is devoted to exploring fundamental epistemological and value issues that form the underpinnings of these concepts.

Twentieth century milestones in the analysis of disease, health and clinical knowledge are French philosopher Georges Canguilhem's 1948/1966 *Le normal et le pathologique* and Michel Foucault's 1963 *La naissance de la clinique*, translated as *The Birth of the Clinic: An Archaeology of Medical Perception*. Foucault's second book, it picks up from *Madness and Civilisation* in its concern with the development and organisation of theoretical and practical knowledge(s) in relation to practices of social organisation. It is a case history, which assembles details that trace the development of the medical profession and clinical knowledge in the institution of the *clinique*, that is, the teaching hospital in Paris at the turn of the nineteenth century. Modern medicine, built on the foundations of the new science of clinical pathology, requires a medical gaze, which closely observes, visually dissects, and instructs. Modern medicine owes the birth of its body of knowledge and practice to the eyes of the doctor.

Foucault's approach to medical discourse is novel, for he is, by and large, not concerned with exclusively medical discourses or a detailed recollection of their history. In *The Birth of the Clinic*, Foucault places medical discourses in a wider network of concerns with, for instance, the health of the population, the training of doctors and shaping of the professional organisation, or regimes of assistance and internment. Foucault's interest is also in the increased concern with the health and welfare of the population and with the process of a noticeable *medicalisation* of society.

Michel Foucault was influenced by Georges Canguilhem's examination of the notions of disease and health *The Normal and the Pathological*. Here, Canguilhem looked at the formation of disease and health in the context of institutions and institutional power. His interest was in the translation of grammatical norms into physiological norms. His exploration into the nature and meaning of normality in medicine and biology, the production and institutionalisation of medical knowledge is still a seminal work in medical philosophy and the history of ideas.

In the 1970s, Anglo-American philosophers started to challenge the dominant positivist ideology of medicine, which discounted personal and cultural evaluation of physical phenomena. This was done on the basis of a growing recognition of the sociology and philosophy of medical knowledge, against the background of

---

19   Von Engelhardt, "History of the Concepts", 1091.

Georges Canguilhem's linking of the relation between health and disease to the requirements of institutional power, and against the backdrop of Michel Foucault's analysis of the development of modern medical epistemology.[20]

Unlike 1960s French philosophy the Anglo-American debate did not focus on power structures or economic and institutional influences on the disease/health distinction but on health in its relation to bodily reality, cultural-dependent values and individually posited life goals. Though in one sense this presents a deficiency in the Anglo-American debate, it is precisely its *exclusive* focus on the themes of body, cultural dependency *or* individuality which makes it central to this study. The Anglo-American interpretations help me show how one-dimensional understandings of health (and human life) have problematic consequences for the physician-patient-relationship as well as for medical practice more widely.

In focusing on the Anglo-American debate, its ancient heritage, and the Church of the first millennium, I will not offer a comprehensive analysis of theological, philosophical or historical attitudes to health and medicine. Even though health and healing are central phenomena in the gospel narratives, I will not offer an in depth historical exegesis of key passages of the New Testament.[21] I will concentrate on the early Church writers, especially Augustine, and the relation of their thought to the contemporary Anglo-American health debate both in the philosophical and theological disciplines.

The study does not engage with medieval philosophy and scholastic theology and its dealings or reservations with medieval medicine.[22] It does not reflect on Thomas Aquinas's considerations on the art of medicine, nature, and human health, such as his view of a co-operation of interior principles of nature and exterior acts committed by the medical agent for the strengthening of nature.[23] It does not inquire into Descartes' anthropology and its mechanical undertones.

Descartes' dualist metaphysics and mechanistic interpretation of matter (not his tentative hints at a psychosomatic dependence or even union) influenced post-Enlightenment anthropologies as well as scientific medicine both methodologically and ontologically.[24] Whilst Cartesianism argued on the basis of a substance dualism, today's materialist philosophers oppose the view that there are two irreducible kinds of things that co-exist. "Materialists uniformly reject Descartes' ontological dualism, in particular, its implication that a human mind is composed of an immaterial substance different in kind from material bodies."[25] For example, the materialism of D. M. Armstrong, one of today's leading materialist philosophers, is largely *monistic* where it insists on all living bodies as nothing but material entities, and where it holds that material things also exemplify psychological

---

20 English translations of both works were available in the mid-1970s.
21 I touch, however, on the New Testament healing stories before looking at the Patristic writers in chapter three.
22 Cf. D.W.Amundsen on medieval medical practice in "Caring and Curing in the Medieval Catholic Tradition" in *Caring and Curing* (1998).
23 Aquinas, *Summa Theologiae*, Question CXVII, First Article.
24 Cf. Lanzerath, *Natürlichkeit der Person*, 95.
25 Moser/Trout, *Contemporary Materialism*, 4–5.

properties and phenomena such as thoughts, beliefs, desires, intentions as well as sensory experiences.

Neither of these philosophical approaches will be given their due attention in this study. This is not to deny their practical relevance or even their influence on contemporary medicine and philosophy of medicine. Yet in focusing on the beginnings of medicine and the bearings these have on the present times, and in seeking a *coherent* conceptual framework for the discussion of health, this study draws above all on Augustine's theology. In understanding the natural body in its personal and social context to be the site of God's love qualified through the life of the Son and restored by the Spirit, both physicians and patients are directed to the horizon of ultimate questions concerned with human striving for fulfilment in the face of mortality. God's care for humanity and his promise of fullness of life in the presence of death are at the heart of Augustine's Christian recognition of medicine. It reveals the art and science of medicine as an essentially legitimate but intrinsically limited means of alleviating pain and restoring health.

The next section provides an outline of the modern philosophical and early Christian understandings of health and medical healing analysed, and of the arguments developed on the basis of this analysis. A brief overview of each chapter is given; references to sub-sections follow in brackets.

1.2 OUTLINE OF ARGUMENTS

Health and disease definitions have practical consequences, and so has any theoretical analysis of them. They are concepts that motivate, guide, shape medical action and health care. They direct health care policies. They are action-guiding concepts. In setting the end for medical action, health and disease are normative concepts. Yet what kind of norm is the norm of health? Is it an absolute norm? Should health be pursued at all costs? Can health trump other moral considerations? Is it a moral virtue? Are we to be held responsible for our health? Are healthy people morally better people?

What *is* health? Illness and disease are more readily and experientially identifiable. They often involve a failure of function, an abnormal pain or the threat of immature death. A negative definition of health identifies it as the absence of disease or deformity, but how can health be defined positively? Is health a description of bodily facts, of empirical data? Or is it a value statement judging physical, social, personal states of existence? The WHO definition, for instance, has been criticised for being too broad and ill defined to guide health policy when it defines health as "a state of complete physical, mental and social well-being and not merely the absence of disease or infirmity". It confuses health with happiness and medicine becomes the sole gatekeeper for human happiness and social well-being.[26]

---

26   It is a good definition in that it acknowledges that there is some intrinsic relationship between the good of the body and the good of the self as well as the wider human community. Yet it is

In order to illustrate how health shapes medical action and policy making, this study begins by looking at the UK policy reports on human embryonic stem cell research and cloning for research.[27] It does not ask substantive questions as to the UK government's understanding of health generally but aims at *illustrating* the role health plays in decision making (health policy decisions being but one example). The chosen documents show health to be central to the conclusion that human embryonic stem cell research and cloning for research is morally permissible and should be legally permitted.

Whilst the reports do *not* reflect explicitly on the *meaning* of health, they attribute value to the *end* of health, even to the mere potential for health. This attribution of value legitimises both medical research action and health policy decisions. Health, then, directs medical and political action. It motivates the promotion of embryonic stem cell research. The reports illustrate the normative power and practical relevance of health.

Before analysing the reports' argumentation, I recapitulate the chronological stages of UK legislation and regulation of assisted reproduction and embryo research. This provides an understanding of the legislative context in which the 1998–2002 debate took place (2.1). Following from here, I detail the reports' arguments in favour of human embryonic stem cell research and analyse how health is connected with a model of balancing values and probabilities (2.2).

In order to address the substantive question as to the meaning of health (not asked in the reports yet crucial given the end of health's normative power) the next chapter goes back to the very beginnings of Western medicine. It engages with second century philosopher and physician Galen, the father of today's medicine. Galen developed an idea of health as the normal or natural state of the body and situated bodily health within the context of the overall striving for welfare, thus combining the two positions. Yet in emphasising the union of body and soul, and the corrective influence of reason or the rational soul, which allows humans to recognise *general* principles for the improvement both of the constitution of the body and the affections of the soul, Galen moves beyond a purely naturalist or individualised welfare account of health. He explicates the need for philosophical education to enable overall human well-being (3.1).

Whilst early Christian writers were interested in Galen's naturalist medicine and in philosophical training, they considered both medicine and philosophy as fragmentary approaches to human life and health, and on this basis as insufficient for well-being or fullness of life. To explore a Christian understanding of human life, and of health, I turn to three early Christian writers: Tatian, a second century Syrian theologian and critic of naturalist medicine; Tertullian, second century theologian of the Latin-speaking West; and Basil the Great, fourth century bishop

---

a problematic definition, to give one example, where it claims health to be the complete state of well-being: the consequence of this would be the total medicalisation of all aspects of human life. See also: Callahan, "The WHO Definition of Health" (1973).

27   The focus is on a selected number of policy reports: an exhaustive account of the *parliamentary* or *public* debate on embryonic research and cloning will not be given in this study.

and Greek-speaking theologian of the East, defender of naturalist medicine. All three thinkers implicitly or explicitly recognise human life as a union of matter and soul. They differ in their views on the causality of disease and health, and the consequences these have for their attitudes towards medical knowledge and practice.

For Tatian diseases of the body are caused by demons, evil forces in nature that act on nature. Healing can be achieved not through naturalist medicine but through the power of God's word which commands the demons to leave the body. Tatian's demonology led him to underestimate the *intrinsic* weakness of bodily nature as potential cause of disease. It also led to his sharp rejection of reason and rationalist medical knowledge, and brought him close to the dualist Gnostic movements of the second century (3.3).

Based on the union of body and soul (which he recognises without explicating it further) Tertullian draws a distinction between physical and spiritual sickness. Spiritual sickness is caused by misguided belief and requires divine cure. Physical diseases may be caused by natural weaknesses of the body, but also by demons. Whilst the former requires knowledge of natural processes, the latter needs the exorcism of demons through the power of the word. Though supporting medical healing, Tertullian's treatment of the sacrament of baptism shows that ultimately spiritual health and healing may lead to eternal flourishing and true human fulfilment (3.4).

In linking diseases and medicine with demons both Tertullian and Tatian are in contrast to Basil the Great. He saw diseases as deficiencies of nature. For him, the body's defective state is related to the Fall not to the influence of demons. Basil supported medical knowledge and practice as an act of charity. He established what was perhaps the West's first hospital. According to Greek Orthodox theologian Stanley Harakas, the views of Basil (as well as Gregory of Nazianzus and Gregory of Nyssa) became the mainline approach of the Greek Orthodox Church towards worldly knowledge, science, and culture (3.5).

Whilst Basil developed his view of medical care from the gospel narratives, in particular the care shown to the sick and underprivileged by Jesus and his apostles, neither he nor his predecessors, Tatian and Tertullian, explicate at length the theological anthropology that underpins their understanding of health and disease.

In chapter four, I turn to St Augustine's theological anthropology which draws together the position of the human creature in body and soul in the world, the understanding of health of body and soul, and the consequences of both for medical practice.

I start with a brief introduction of Augustine's view on creation and the Creator, which explains human life as both given and in *a priori* relationship with its Creator. Augustine speaks about creation not as a scientific process but as the beginning of existence through God's will. Created existence according to God's word is *good* and *ordered*. Created bodies exist in a hierarchical order of relationships, which originates in the relational love of the Trinitarian God.[28] This irrevocably attributes value to the whole that is creation and to all its parts (4.1).

Human existence is material and bodily, yet it is never the life of the body only. The body-soul union is central to Augustine's anthropology. Humans are composite beings, not bodies nor souls alone but body and soul together. The biblical doctrine of the resurrection confirms the union of body and soul: here the body is taken up into eternity and remains the very same, particular body (*my* body or *your* body). Together with the incarnation, the resurrection affirms the goodness of the body. Augustine shows that the incarnation and resurrection are the foundation of the Christian understanding of the goodness of the human body and of God's claim upon the human body (4.2).

Whilst recognising the goodness of the body, Augustine holds that the soul is the creature's superior part which not only animates, but also dominates the body. I inquire with key Augustinian scholars as to Augustine's understanding of the human soul in the context of the *imago Dei* doctrine. Augustine understands God's image, that is, goodness and love, to be inalienably located in the human soul. Here, God relates to humans, who in turn desire to relate to him: what is more natural then to love *love*?[29] The *imago Dei*, hence, indicates the relationship between the Creator and the creature, and from there between all God's creatures. The *imago* constitutes the intrinsically *personal* dimension of human life (a human being is the particular *you* of God's loving address), as well as its *social* dimension, its being directed to the other (who is also addressed as *you*). It qualifies the attitude humans should have both towards themselves and to each other as an attitude of *love*.

I will look closely at three particular aspects of Augustine's interpretation of the *imago*, namely, the relational, dynamic, proleptic aspects, which have implications for his view of health, as well as medical healing and medical morality.

I will also look at Augustine's interpretation of the Fall. Due to the Fall, the image of God's love in humans is discoloured and in need of renewal or restoration brought to humans in Christ and mediated by the Spirit (4.3).

Though Augustine resolutely defended the goodness of matter, he was also painfully aware of the deficiencies of nature which humans experience most acutely in bodily illness and in the encounter with death. He understands evil in nature (e.g. diseases) as God's punishment for the freely chosen disobedience in the Garden. Such punishment for Augustine is just and inherited. It functions as an exhortation to the conversion of people's hearts to God's love. God's salvific love is the primary context in which Augustine reflected on human health and (medical) healing (4.4).

Bodily health is a gift of grace which belongs to the history of human salvation. It reflects God's end for humanity which is happiness, joy, and well-being. God extends being, and gives well-being, temporal here and now, and perfect in the future. Augustine saw medicine as one possible means of healing. God's

---

28 Augustine, *City of God*, XI/10.
29 Augustine, *Trinity*, VIII/10.

mercy and grace works in the medical profession but God is also known to have healed in the sacrament of baptism and in response to prayer (4.5).

Like Tertullian, Augustine distinguished disease and health of body and soul. Illness of the soul is a result of humanity's separation from God after the Fall. This separation leads to love of self, instead of love of God, and behaviour such as lust, envy or greed. The full restoration of the *imago* (hence, of the creature's relationship to God, self, and the other) is not a sudden and immediate event. It is a gradual process, which takes place during one's lifetime and will be completed eschatologically. Healing of the soul needs to be striven for first, in remitting the cause in baptism, and second, in orienting one's *self* to the love of God and meeting others on this basis. The soul's health is valued higher than all bodily health: it leads the human creature in its union of body and soul to the fullness of love (4.6).

Chapter five focuses on the Anglo-American debate from the mid-1970s. Against the background of the unitive account of Augustine I will explicate the impact that an isolated reflection on the body, or the individual, or the social context may have on medical practice. At the centre of the 1970s debate was the question whether health and disease are natural norms shared by all members of the human species (with the exception of a few disease anomalies) or whether they are standards underpinned by value judgments and imposed on individuals in a particular socio-political context. At present, the debate is heading towards theories that seek to bridge natural-factual and socio-cultural-evaluative aspects of health and disease, and situates health increasingly in the context of human flourishing (5.1).

After an introductory overview, I look at the American naturalist philosopher Christopher Boorse for whom health is a statistical norm. Health and disease are a matter of empirical investigation: medicine reads off symptoms of bodily functioning and dysfunctioning. Whilst giving health a clear epistemological status, Boorse's approach reduces the meaning of health to bodily functionality. The body is seen as an isolated natural entity, separate from e.g. individual choices, opinions, emotions or desires. On a practical level, this means that the body, like a material object, may be handed over to the physician (5.2).

H. Tristram Engelhardt (here in his role as a medical philosopher) acknowledged that concepts of disease and health include empirical bodily parameters yet rejected Boorse's purely naturalist account. Using the example of the nineteenth century disease of masturbation, Engelhardt argued for a value-infected and culture-dependent concept of health. In raising awareness for the impact of cultural or political norms on decisions of what state of human life or what human actions are considered to be signs of health or disease, Engelhardt's evaluative understanding allowed for deconstructing the physician's assumed neutrality and authority. However, in focusing on the social and cultural context primarily, he failed to explore the individual component in interpreting the concept of health against, for instance, the horizon of one's personal life-experience and hopes for a fulfilled future (5.3).

Lennart Nordenfelt's account of health focuses on the individual dimension of human life in relation to health. For him, health is a state of life that allows us to achieve our vital goals. These result from individual choices. As a consequence, there are as many healths as there are individual assumptions, beliefs, propositions, and choices. Nordenfelt's interpretation allows medicine and health care more generally to centre on the subjective needs and desires of the patient, and to enable his or her goal achievements. Yet the question remains whether a common (social, cultural, political or indeed natural) underpinning of health can be recognised in such subjective interpretations. A common reference point is important as basis of shared health care systems and codes of professional conduct (5.4).

The final chapter draws out conclusions for the physician-patient relationship and medical practice developed on the basis of an Augustinian understanding of human life and health in critical comparison with contemporary philosophical accounts of health.

The exegesis of theologians of the past with a view to their relevance for today's medical practices is undertaken together with an exploration of twentieth and twenty-first century theological discourse on health and the relationship between theology and medicine. Why might the study of a theologian or theologians of the past be important for debating medical morality today? For today's Orthodox theologians with their understanding of the workings of the Spirit in the present the theological predecessors of the first millennium are contemporaries.[30]

For today's Western theologians God's revelation in Christ and in Scripture and the tradition, in varying degrees according to various traditions, is not only an historical event, but is present in the church always.

In chapter six I engage with Karl Barth's views on abundant human life, health, medicine, and the relationship of the individual to God and fellow humans. I look at H. Tristram Engelhardt's work, writing now as Orthodox Christian bioethicist on issues of bodily and spiritual health and the rich Orthodox tradition of miraculous healing. I explore Stanley Hauerwas' views on the importance of the church for medical practice as a community able to be present to others in pain.

I seek to bring out how the positions of the Church Fathers presented above, and Augustine's views in particular, accord with the interpretations and views offered by our contemporaries. Against this argumentative background I will move on to develop an approximation of how health might be understood in the contemporary context when approached from a perspective that seeks to take seriously the wisdom found in the engagement with God's word in Scripture and the Christian tradition (6.1).

Grounded in Augustine's anthropology which integrates body and soul, bodily health is recognised as a component of human ontology; patients share the physical and physiological generalities of a species. Yet in facing a particular patient, the physician faces a unique person with an inimitable life story, the knowledge and interpretation of which can be decisive for success of treatment – an aspect that belongs to her ontology also. Where the body is good, its state of health is *a good*. Yet when particular practices of medical research and/or clinical treatment convey an understanding of health and healing that fails to acknowledge the ontology of the body as integrating personal particularities as is the case in the UK documents' rhetoric of repair, these practices cease to be oriented towards the good of human health which the exegesis of Augustine's anthropology developed.

Bodily health is a *temporal* and *relative* good. It is a *temporal* good due to the body's temporal finitude; it is a *relative* good measured against God's absolute love. Health's temporal nature and relative value limits medical research and clinical action against the horizon of finitude and, above all, infinite being. Where health is recognised as a state that serves human life in its orientation towards God's being, health may motivate medical action. Then, it may indeed function as a research imperative and promote medical action.

2. ILLUSTRATING THE NORMATIVE FUNCTION OF HEALTH: UK STEM CELL POLICIES

Human *embryonic* stem cell research is a comparatively recent area of research. Whilst *human* stem cell research has existed for about 20 years, the first success in the isolation and culture of human pluripotent *embryonic* stem cells dates back only to 1998.[31] Until then most embryonic stem cell research was dependent on animal models, mainly mouse models. In 1984, Lady Warnock's Report on embryo research stated: "Although many research studies in embryology and developmental biology can be carried out on animal subjects, and it is possible in many cases to extrapolate these results and findings to man, in certain situations there is no substitute for the use of human embryos."[32] Indeed, there are certain disorders such as Down's syndrome which only occur in humans. Also, the process of human fertilisation as well as some specific effects of drugs on human tissue can only be studied in humans.[33] Hence, medical research requires *human* embryos and *human* embryonic stem cells where it seeks to inquire into species-specific development and diseases.

Embryonic stem cell research makes possible the study of embryonic development more generally, and in particular of the processes of differentiation and de-differentiation of cells. Experimentation upon embryonic stem cells increases the understanding of how, in the process of the formation of the complete organism, embryonic cells differentiate into the mature cells that give rise to functional units. At the same time, embryonic stem cell research provides insights into the molecular nature of normal and abnormal cell organisation, development, growth, maturation, and ageing processes. It advances general knowledge of cell processes.

The United Kingdom has been at the forefront of the rapidly growing area of stem cell research and the related field of cloning.[34] Human embryonic stem cell research with its therapeutic potential is considered a major economic growth

---

31 Thomson, "Embryonic Stem Cell Lines", 1145–1147.
32 Warnock, *Question of Life*, 62.
33 Ibid.
34 During the 1980s, Sir Martin Evans and his team in Cambridge pioneered stem cell science in studies of mice; in Edinburgh in 1997, Prof. Ian Wilmut and his team showed how cloning could be used to turn back adult body cells into versatile embryonic stem cells. In 2004, the United Kingdom became one of the first nations to permit the creation of human embryos through cloning techniques for embryonic stem cell research. Two licences have been awarded for therapeutic cloning: to the Newcastle Fertility Centre at Life (www.nfc-life.com, last accessed 12/09), and jointly to the Roslin Institute in Edinburgh and King's College London. In 2005, the UK was able to announce its first successfully cloned human embryo (Newcastle University team around Prof. Alison Murdoch).

area.[35] As part of the wider area of stem cell research, it benefits from the large amounts of public money invested in the general research field.

In March 2005 the UK Government established the UK Stem Cell Initiative charged with developing a cohesive vision for UK stem cell research for the coming ten years.[36] The Initiative, which published its first report in November 2005, suggests that "*the ultimate health and wealth gains* that the UK will enjoy are directly proportional to the proposed additional investment."[37] The UK Government set up the world's first stem cell bank hosted by the National Institute for Biological Standards and Control (NIBSC). This bank is a repository for stem cells of all types, that is, adult, foetal, and embryonic, and supplies cell lines both for research and applications (where available). At the time of its opening, the NIBSC website emphasised the bank's commitment "to working closely with researchers, clinicians, funding bodies, industry and regulators, *to bring this major opportunity for improving human health to fruition.*"[38]

Both the UK Stem Cell Initiative and the UK Stem Cell Bank as beneficiaries of state investment are keen to underline "health gains" as major incentive for the promotion of stem cell research as a primary area of medical research. To illustrate how the end of health guides action not only in medical practice and research but also in health policy making, I look at the 1998–2002 UK policy reports on human embryonic stem cell research and cloning for research.[39]

I have chosen these documents for three reasons: (1) The 1998–2002 policy initiative was politically successful. It led to the revision of existing legislation on embryonic research and created the legislative framework that allowed the subsequent advances in UK embryonic stem cell research to take place. (2) Emphasis on the *goal of health* was central to its success. Unanimously, the reports conclude that human embryonic stem cell research and cloning for research should be legally permitted because of its therapeutic potential. (3) Focusing on a morally

35   According to the scientific community, the derivation of pluripotent stem cells from adult body cells by Japanese researchers in 2007 does not call into question research on embryonic stem cells. Induced pluripotent stem cells (iPS cells) are derived artificially from a non-pluripotent somatic cell by inducing a number of genes – a method, which in the meantime has been reproduced by various research teams around the globe.
      In a 2010 interview with the *Times* Sir Ian Wilmut emphasised that „ES cells remained the gold standard" despite stem cells technology's rapid advances (www.timesonline.co.uk/tol/-news/uk/scotland/article7076659.ece, last accessed 04/2010).
      See also e.g. the Berlin-Brandenburg Academy of the Sciences (BBAW) 2010 *Zweiter Gentechnologiebericht* which emphasises the need for parallel research on adult, embryonic and induced stem cells (chapter two).
36   See http://www.dh.gov.uk/ab/UKSCI/index.htm, last accessed 01/2010.
37   The *2005 Report & Recommendations* of the UK Stem Cell Initiative are available at http://www.dh.gov.uk/ab/UKSCI/index.htm, last accessed 01/2010 (my italics).
38   At the time of the UK stem cell bank's opening in 2005, this information was available at www.nibsc.ac.uk/spotlight/ukstemcell.html (last accessed 11/2005, my italics). The UK stem cell bank's own website is http://www.ukstemcellbank.org.uk/, last accessed 01/2010.
39   In focusing on policy reports, a comprehensive account of the *parliamentary* or *public* debate on embryonic research and cloning and their notions of health or disease will not be provided here.

contentious field of research and the documents that reflect and capture the decision making process, allows me to highlight how powerful the goal 'health' is in solving moral quandaries. The documents illustrate how health was used to trump other moral considerations and action-guiding principles such as for instance the prohibition of taking human life.

Clearly, embryonic stem cell research with its claims for an improvement of human health, on which political and societal support is founded, is but *one* aspect of a technology dominated culture. Yet as an area where controversy abounds and moral debates are fought, it is an area that can aptly illustrate the power health exercises in the contemporary societal context. And where the goal of health plays such a crucial role in solving moral quandaries, questions as to its meaning – how is health understood? How can it be understood? Should it be understood in one particular way or is there a plurality of health? – are highly relevant. Hence, the chapter before us functions as a gateway to the reflection of the notion of health which is at the heart of this study. It does so by underlining the relevance of a conceptual analysis for moral debate in contemporary medicine and by illustrating the power that health in fact exercises in decision-making processes.

This chapter, then, does not ask how health is understood *generally*. I will not look at documents such as the Department of Health's 1998 Green Paper *Our Healthier Nation* or the 2004 White Paper *Choosing Health*.[40] Whilst both show the importance given to public health in contemporary political culture, they do not provide us with cases that illustrate the power the end of health exercises in debates on the morality of particular avenues of medical research.

Apart from Lady Warnock's 1984 Report as key reference both for legislation and policy documents, this chapter's main primary resources are the 1998 Human Fertilisation and Embryology Authority/Human Genetics Advisory Commission's joint report on *Cloning Issues in Reproduction, Science and Medicine: A Consultation Document*; the 2000 Department of Health's report on *Stem Cell Research: Medical Progress with Responsibility. A Report from the Chief Medical Officer's Expert Group Reviewing the Potential of Developments in Stem Cell Research and Cell Nuclear Replacement to Benefit Human Health* as well as the UK Government's *Response to the Recommendations Made in the Chief Medical Officer's*

---

40   What is more, the 1998 and 2004 government documents do not attempt a definition of health, and have little *directly* to say about the meaning of health. The definition of health implied by the documents is of health as physical and mental well-being, which is directly influenced by our behaviour in that we make certain lifestyle choices. Social influences (living and working conditions, job security and so on) are recognised, too. Yet generally, health in our democratic societies is described as based on our choices: where we choose not to smoke or drink alcohol, where we exercise regularly, and eat plenty of fruit and vegetables, we are opting for health or better: a healthy lifestyle. "Health improvement depends upon people's motivation and their willingness to act on it. The Government will provide information and practical support to get people motivated and improve emotional wellbeing and access to services so that healthy choices are easier to make" (7). This view of health as 'our option' is interesting in so far as disease, which is often defined as the symmetrical opposite of health – also in the documents on embryonic stem cell research – is mostly experienced as a condition that befalls us and is outside human choosing, outside human volition.

Expert Group Report 'Stem Cell Research: Medical Progress with Responsibility' and the House of Lords Select Committee's 2002 report on *Stem Cell Research: Report from the Select Committee.*

2.1 EMBRYONIC RESEARCH: LEGISLATION AND REGULATION

The UK Parliament passed the Human Fertilisation and Embryology Act twenty years ago.[41] The Act focuses on embryo research, welfare of the child, and abortion. It resulted from debates on issues surrounding reproductive technologies, fertilisation, parenthood and embryo research which peaked around 1978 when Louise Brown was born, the first birth resulting from the use of *in vitro* fertilisation (IVF).

Largely, the HFE Act followed the recommendations of Lady Warnock's committee, which inquired into options for infertility treatment, appropriate policies and safeguards. The committee was set up by the UK Government in 1982 to direct attention not only to future practices of fertility treatment and possible legislation, "but to the principles on which such practices and such legislation would rest."[42] It published its report in July 1984 (the Warnock Report).[43] Questions around the morality of cloning for research purposes were not yet on the agenda.

Mary Warnock, a moral philosopher, chaired the 16-member committee, which was dominated by medical scientists and health professionals.[44] Members of the committee wanted "to attempt to discover the public good, in the widest sense, and to make recommendations in the light of that."[45] Accordingly, the committee's recommendations for legislation sought to embody "a common moral position" and "a broad framework for what is morally acceptable within society."[46] The committee explicitly rejected a utilitarian position mainly for its inability to take into account the "strong sentiments"[47] which the committee members encountered throughout the process of evidence gathering.

After introducing the field of embryo research and briefly surveying the biological causes and psychological effects of childlessness and the services available to infertile couples in chapter two, the Warnock Report devotes seven out of its 13

---

41   HFE Act 1990 (c.37): www.hmso.gov.uk/acts/acts1990/Ukpga_19900037_en_1.htm, last accessed 01/2010. The HFEA Act was updated in 2008 with the amendments coming into force on 1st October 2009. The statutory storage period for embryos was changed from 5 to 10 years (cf. also http://www.hfea.gov.uk/371.html, last accessed 01/2010). These amendments do not affect the argument pursued here.

42   Warnock, *Question of Life*, 1.

43   M. Warnock, *A Question of Life: the Warnock Report on Human Fertilisation and Embryology with two New Chapters* (London, 1985).

44   For a full list of the members of the Warnock Committee, see Warnock, *Question of Life*, iv–v.

45   Warnock, *Question of Life*, 1.

46   Ibid., 3.

47   Ibid., 2.

chapters to the discussion of services such as artificial insemination, *in vitro* ferti-lisation, egg donation, embryo donation, and surrogacy. It has a particular focus on three ethical issues which it says are common to all these services: anonymity, counselling, and consent.[48] The possible uses of embryos in scientific research are discussed in chapter eleven. The Report finishes with an overview of possible future developments in fertility treatment and research (this includes cloning) in chapter twelve and regulation recommendations in chapter thirteen. Here, the es-tablishment of a new statutory licensing body is suggested as a priority.[49]

A key conclusion of Lady Warnock's committee is that the human embryo prior to fourteen days of development has a "special status" entitling it to some protection in law. Concretely, the committee recommended that research may not be undertaken except on embryos prior to fourteen days of development and under a licence issued by the regulatory body. The embryo's special moral status in con-nection with the fourteen-day-limit is considered a firm foundation for legislation on assisted reproduction, embryo research, and cloning to the present day.[50]

The Warnock Report led the way to the Human Fertilisation and Embryology Act 1990. In accordance with the concerns of the time, the Act regulates the prac-tice of in vitro fertilisation (IVF) and the creation, use, storage and disposal of embryos formed in the process of IVF treatment. It is

"An act to make provision in connection with human embryos and any subsequent develop-ment of such embryos; to prohibit certain practices in connection with embryos and gametes; to establish a Human Fertilisation and Embryology Authority."[51]

The act largely implements the recommendations of Mary Warnock's report, for instance, where it states that any research on embryos older than fourteen days or after the appearance of the primitive streak (whichever is the earliest) is prohi-bited.[52] Any research prior to fourteen days may not be undertaken except under a licence issued by the Human Fertilisation and Embryology Authority (HFEA),[53] a statutory body established under section 5 of the Act.[54] The UK licensing system is unique; no other country has a regulatory agency which centres on the human embryo.

---

48 Warnock, *Question of Life*, 15.
49 Ibid., 80–86.
50 The Warnock Committee's approach regarding the moral status of the embryo and the 14-day-limit has been endorsed more recently by the House of Common's Science & Technol-ogy Committee, Human Reproductive Technologies and the Law, 5th Report of session 2004–05, 28 (16); 46 (22); 58 (29). The approach has been confirmed by the UK Government in its Response to the Report (August 2005), 8(7); 15(9).
51 HFE Act 1990.
52 Ibid., 3.(3)–(4).
53 Ibid., 3. (1).
54 Ibid., 5. (1)–(3).

Under Schedule 2 of the Act a licence may not be granted "unless the Authority is satisfied that any proposed use of embryos is necessary for the purposes of the research"[55] and

"Cannot authorise any activity unless it appears to the Authority to be necessary or desirable for the purposes of: (a) promoting advances in the treatment of infertility, (b) increasing knowledge about the causes of congenital disease, (c) increasing knowledge about the causes of miscarriages, (d) developing more effective techniques of contraception, (e) developing methods for detecting the presence of gene or chromosome abnormalities in embryos before implantation, or for such other purposes as may be specified in regulations."[56]

A peer-review committee considers applications for research licences and assesses whether the proposed research falls under the permitted purposes and whether it is necessary for achieving the permitted purposes. After an interim period which saw the foundation of the Voluntary Licensing Authority for human in vitro Fertilisation and Embryology (VLA) in 1985, the Human Fertilisation and Embryology Authority (HFEA)[57] was formed and took up its full statutory responsibility in 1991. The HFEA is a

"Non-departmental Government body that regulates and inspects all UK clinics providing IVF, donor insemination or the storage of eggs, sperm or embryos. The HFEA also licenses and monitors all human embryo research being conducted in the UK."[58]

This includes regulation of the creation, storage, and use of embryos for research. While the 1990 Act contains a number of prohibitions on the uses of human embryos, it gives wide powers of interpretation to the HFEA.[59] Numerous scientific developments have taken place since 1990, which have led to a number of revisions of the 1990 Act. For instance, the storage period for gametes (1991) and frozen embryos (1996) was extended, and reproductive cloning (2001) was prohibited.[60] The question of how to interpret the meaning of the term embryo has

---

55   HFE Act 1990, Schedule 2, 3 (6).
56   Ibid., Schedule 2, 3 (2).
57   See http://www.hfea.gov.uk/Home, last accessed 01/2010.
58   Ibid.
59   For an overview of currently approved research projects see: http://www.hfea.gov.uk/166.-html, last accessed 01/2010.
60   For an overview of all revisions, see House of Commons Science & Technology Committee, Human reproductive Technologies and the Law, 5th Report of session 2004–05, Table 2, 9. In response to the rapid medical and scientific progress and in light of European and other international legislation and treatises, on 21 January 2004 the Department of Health announced a general review of the HFE Act, in the process of which it is consulting the public (Review of the Human Fertilisation and Embryology Act, A Public Consultation, DoH 2005), and looking to the House of Commons Science & Technology Committee's Inquiry on Human Reproductive Technologies and the Law (24.03.2005). Though this review, which passed parliament in 2008 and came into effect in 2009, changed existing legislation, it did not address embryo stem cell research and the creation of embryos for research purposes (see S&T Committee 5th Report, chapter three and seven). In fact, the Department of Health's review of the 1990 Act explicitly excluded the 1990–2002 policy and parliamentary debate.

been at the centre of the debate so far.[61] In 2005, the Human Tissue Authority (HTA) was established under the 2004 Human Tissue Act as an executive non-departmental body sponsored by the Department of Health. While the HFEA continues to deal with embryos, the HTA regulates the keeping of cell lines derived from embryos.

> "Once a line has been created it is a condition of an HFEA research licence that a sample line is deposited in the UK Stem Cell Bank. At this point, the HFEA's regulatory remit ceases. The HTA's regulatory authority commences at the point the embryo is disorganised and cells are grown to create cell lines with the intention that the lines may at some future time be used in human application. Therefore, any organisation, processing, testing, storing, and distributing of cell lines with the intention that they may be used in human application may (since July 5th 2007), only do so under the authority of an HTA licence."[62]

2.2 POLICY DOCUMENTS ON EMBRYONIC STEM CELL RESEARCH

Potential health benefits are key to an understanding of much of the attraction of human embryonic stem cell research not only for the scientific research community but also for policy makers with their predominant interest in the electorate's perception of being benefited. The three main policy documents that initiated, accompanied and followed the 2000/2001 parliamentary debates on human embryonic stem cell research unanimously claim that potential health benefits are perhaps the primary motivation for pursuing this avenue of research.

The moral dilemma that the three documents face is that human embryonic stem cell research involves the destruction of the human embryo prior to fourteen days of development. Can such destruction be morally justified? In answering this question, the documents use stem cell research's therapeutic potential to respond to concerns about the status of the embryo. For a definition of the embryo's status all three documents refer to the 1984 Warnock Report and its interpretation of the beginning of personhood after fourteen days of development.

The section's overall aim is neither to analyse a particular case of health policy making nor to offer an in-depth exploration of the meaning of health as tentatively implied in the documents. Its aim is more simply to illustrate that the end of health is practically relevant for policy decisions and medical research, and that therefore a reflection as to its meaning is not only an academic issue but is of practical relevance, and that therefore all subsequent theoretical reflection on health may be assessed in light of its practical consequences.

---

61 For an overview of the significant legal cases surrounding the HFE Act, see House of Commons Science & Technology Committee, Human reproductive Technologies and the Law, 5th Report of session 2004–05, Table 3, 10.
62 See https://www.hta.gov.uk (last accessed 01/2010). The HTA also ensures that research conforms to the requirements of the EUTCD (European Tissue and Cells Directive).

2.2.1 The 1984 Warnock Report

The embryo is *alive* where its cells divide and develop. This is beyond debate. Yet the question of its personhood is known to be controversial. It demands regulation and legislation on a national and even international level. Is the embryo a person? If so, it has rights, and presumably the most fundamental of all rights: the right to life. In this, the question of personhood is not only controversial but also critical. As American medical ethicist Richard McCormick remarks: "It is critical because it may determine what we conclude is morally appropriate or inappropriate to do with pre-embryos."[63]

According to Lady Warnock's committee, questions as to whether or not the human embryo is indeed a human being are "complex amalgams of factual and moral judgements."[64] In chapter eleven, the report lists some of the key arguments against and for the use of embryos in research which are centred on the beginning of life and/or personhood (11.11–11.15) and then goes straight onto the question "of *how it is right to treat the human embryo.*"[65] It assesses the *legal* situation of the human embryo in the United Kingdom and concludes that whilst a measure of protection is provided "the human embryo *per se* has no legal status. It is not, under law in the United Kingdom accorded the same status as a child or an adult and the law does not treat the human embryo as having a right to life."[66]

Nevertheless, amongst the population, the committee continues, the more generally held position[67] is "that the embryo of the human species ought to have a special status and that no one should undertake research on human embryos the purposes of which could be achieved by the use of other animals or in some other way."[68] Thus it recommends that the human embryo "should be afforded some protection in law"[69] and "that research conducted on human *in vitro* embryos and the handling of such embryos should be permitted only under licence."[70] On this the committee agrees when it concludes with a majority vote that research on human embryos should continue, though under clear regulation.[71]

However, the question the committee still needs to tackle is what "some protection in law" means in practice, for instance with regard to the time limit on keeping human *in vitro* embryos alive for research (11.20–11.21). This includes

---

63 McCormick, "Who or What is the Pre-embryo", 8. 'Pre-embryo' is the term which McCormick prefers for scientific reasons (his words) because it still contains cells which will later form the placenta and umbilical cord, hence, are not the embryo proper. Biologically, however, such distinction seems only partially correct: we speak of the 'whole fruit' as being contained within the embryonic sac; also birth is only considered complete once the placenta is delivered.

64 Warnock, *Question of Life*, 60.

65 Ibid.

66 Ibid., 62.

67 Ibid.

68 Ibid., 63.

69 Ibid.

70 Ibid., 64.

71 Ibid.

the following questions: up to what point in their development should embryos be granted what the Warnock Report calls special status? When do they acquire the status of a child or an adult and become entitled to more than special status, namely to absolute respect and protection in law?

As possible answers to these questions, the Warnock committee lists different positions such as the capacity to feel pain at about 22 or 23 days after fertilisation,[72] or early neural development at 14 days.[73] It recommends, as limit on keeping embryos alive, the beginning of the embryo's individual development which coincides with the appearance of the primitive streak at around 14 days of development.[74] The primitive streak *marks* the development of individuality in that it takes place at about fourteen days *post* fertilisation which is the latest stage at which twinning events can occur (11.5). This also coincides with the process of implantation, which in most cases is completed at around the fourteenth day so that the fourteen-day limit "is consonant with the views of those who favour the end of the implantation stage as a limit."[75]

On the basis of such understanding of embryonic development, the Warnock committee's conclusion is that up to the fourteenth day, or after the primitive streak has been formed, a human embryo should be granted special value status in law.[76] Up to the fourteenth day of development an embryo can be kept alive and research can be permitted under the control and monitoring from the HFEA as licensing body. After fourteen days the *in vitro* embryo is to be accorded absolute respect. It may not be used in research no matter how beneficial the research may promise to be.[77]

Special status, then, is a value status different to that of a child or adult (who are both full human beings) and different to that of other human cells and tissue (which have no potential of developing into a human being) as well as different to that of a mouse and other animals (which are other species altogether). The embryo is granted moral value because it is *human*. Yet the degree of its value depends on a particular ontological status: its being a human *individual*.

The embryo's value is relative to the process of individual development. It is of special value prior to fourteen days (where twinning events can still occur) and it is of absolute value post fourteen days when it is marked as one, or two, individual(s). The degree of respect owed to the embryo depends on (a) the species and (b) the embryo's individual development. For the Report, special respect is not an ontological downgrading, as it were. On the contrary, the impression is that respect and status have been granted to the embryo at fourteen days on the basis of its ontological (developmental) status.

72 Warnock, *Question of Life*, 65.
73 Ibid.
74 Ibid., 66.
75 Ibid.
76 Ibid., 62.
77 An unsolved issue is that the embryo post-fourteen days is in fact accorded *no* respect when it is discarded where not used in research, not transferred to a uterus or not cryo-conserved in the process of IVF procedures.

The fourteen days mark as cut-off point has become the foundation of embryonic research legislation in the United Kingdom. Apart from the policy documents a more recent affirmation of the fourteen day rule can be found in the House of Commons' Science and Technology Committee's 2004–05 Report on *Human Reproductive Technologies and the Law*. The Report states:

> "We have been told that the 14 day rule is an arbitrary cut off point. For many, even those who support assisted reproduction and embryo research, an extension to the 14-day rule would be unacceptable. We accept that there is *no case at present for an extension, or indeed reduction*. However, we believe that, if scientists or clinicians were able to provide convincing justification for any change, this should be determined by Parliament."[78]

Having introduced the view of the embryo's value status, which is key to the three policy reports, I now turn to these documents. In looking at the 1998 HFEA/HGAC Report, the 2000 CMO Report and the 2002 HoL Select Committee Report, I will draw out the references made to health and how health trumps other ends of medical practice and research.

2.2.2 The 1998 HFEA/HGAC Consultation document

An extension of the five purposes of embryonic research as set up in the 1990 HFE Act was first considered in 1998 by the HFEA and the Human Genetics Advisory Commission (HGAC), a non-statutory advisory body, now the Human Genetics Commission (HGC). Both argued,

> "When the 1990 HFE Act was passed, the beneficial therapeutic consequences that could potentially result from human embryo research were not envisaged."[79]

By "beneficial therapeutic consequences" both bodies had in mind treatment for cell-based diseases or injuries. The aim was to extend the research purposes set up in the 1990 Act beyond research into, and the treatment of, infertility. Wider therapeutic applications should be made possible. The two commissioning bodies understood that research into cell-based therapies would benefit from cloning of embryos for research: stem cells extracted from an embryonic clone of one's own body prevent immune rejection reactions. For this reason, the commissions' public consultation exercise focused almost entirely on cloning as the most contested moral issue in embryonic research. The purpose of the consultation "was not to reopen old debates"[80] about the HFE Act but to consider "the effectiveness of the Act in dealing with new developments concerning cloning."[81]

The HFEA/HGAC joint statement *Cloning Issues in Reproduction, Science and Medicine* reported on the 1998 public consultation exercise. In sections two and eight it reflects on public worries. Further, it reviews the legal and administrative context of embryo research and cloning in the UK and internationally (sec-

---

78   STC, 5th Report, 58, 29 (my italics).
79   HGAC/HFEA, *Cloning Issues*, 9.3., 32.
80   Ibid., 9.1., 32.
81   Ibid.

tions three and seven) and reflects on the potential therapeutic benefits of scientific developments in reproductive medicine, embryo research, and cloning (sections four and five). Annex C offers a summary analysis of responses. The HGAC/HFEA hoped that their report would "contribute to improved understanding of the issues around human cloning and nuclear transfer technology, and how they might best be addressed in the future." Wide potential benefits of the technology of cloning for stem cell research should be maximised, while at the same time concerns needed to be recognised and adequate safeguards implemented.[82]

The terms *clone* and *cloning* carry a stigma and inspire worries, angst and hype, HGAC and HGC observe. For the non-scientific community cloning is met with strong, mainly intuitive resistance as it "carries an automatic stigma for many because of its association with imagery such as that portrayed in Brave New World."[83] This might seem surprising, in that clones occur *in* nature (regularly at least in lower organisms which reproduce asexually but also, one could argue, in higher organisms as in the case of identical twins in humans), and cloning *of* natural organisms is a traditional and widely used technique of agriculture or horticulture. Yet human instincts seem to strongly go against artificially produced clones of their own species.

The 1998 HGAC/HFEA report refers to the technique of cloning as "cell nucleus replacement" or the "therapeutic use of cell nucleus replacement."[84] "To avoid confusion"[85] with reproductive cloning (which is widely considered morally impermissible[86]), this terminological proposition describes both action (cell nucleus replacement) and aim (therapeutic use) but avoids naming the action's product (the cloned human embryo). The term focuses on technical procedures and their possible benefits for sufferers from cell-based diseases. This can help, the Report suggests, in convincing the lay community. Research cloning does not aim to produce designer babies but to gain "immunologically compatible tissues for the *treatment* of degenerative diseases of, for example, the heart, liver, kidneys and cerebral tissue, or *repair* damage to skin or bone."[87]

Against the background of health benefits, in the concluding section nine HGAC/HFEA recommend two further purposes of embryo research for which licences might be issued by the HFEA. Both purposes would usefully involve the

---

82 HGAC/HFEA, *Cloning Issues,* Foreword, 2.
83 Ibid., 5.1, 19.
84 Ibid., section 5 (heading) and 5.1, 19.
85 Ibid.
86 UNESCO's 1997 Declaration on the Human Genome and Human Rights, Article 11 ("Practices which are contrary to human dignity, such as reproductive cloning of human beings, shall not be permitted.") at www.portal.unesco.org, last accessed 04/2010. In a similar vein see also the more recent report on the ethical issues of human cloning (published in 2004 at http://unesdoc.unesco.org/images/0013/001359/135928e.pdf, last accessed 04/2010). The Council of Europe 1997 Convention on human rights and biomedicine, additional protocol on the prohibition of cloning human beings, article 1 ("Any intervention seeking to create a human being genetically identical to another human being, whether living or dead, is prohibited") http://conventions.coe.int/treaty/en/treaties/html/168.htm, last accessed 04/2010.
87 HGAC/HFEA, *Cloning Issues,* 5.6, 21 (my italics).

cloning of embryos. Both are considered therapeutic in intention in so far as they are concerned with (a) the development of "methods of therapy for mitochondrial diseases" and (b) the development of "methods of therapy for diseased or damaged tissues or organs."[88] To extend the five existing purposes for which the HFEA might issue licences for research would mean "potential benefits" of embryonic stem cell research "can clearly be explored."[89]

2.2.3 The 2000 Chief Medical Officer's Report

In 1999, following the HGAC/HFEA Report and its recommendations for an extension of research purposes the Government set up an expert group under the chairmanship of the then Chief Medical Officer (CMO), Prof. Liam Donaldson.

"The Group was asked to undertake an assessment of the anticipated benefits of new areas of research using human embryos, the risks and alternatives, and in the light of that assessment, to advise whether these new areas of research should be permitted."[90]

The group published its report in June 2000.[91] Under the headings "Cells for research and treatment" the CMO Report provided an overview of the techniques "which could yield cells capable of repairing diseased or damaged organs."[92]

It considered some of the scientific and technical problems (chapter two: "The possibilities"), set out the "legal framework governing the use of embryos in research"[93] (chapter three: "Legal considerations"), and discussed some of "the major concerns about stem cell technology"[94] (chapter four: "Ethical considerations"; note that the discussion of ethical considerations takes place after the health benefits of scientific developments have been established[95]).

The CMO Report reviews scientific evidence and recommends research using embryos created by either *in vitro* fertilisation or *somatic cell nucleus replacement* (SCNR) that is, cloning. It repeats that reproductive cloning is "ethically unacceptable and [...] cannot happen in this country."[96] It is aware that therapeutic cloning as a term has led to much confusion in that it links positive and negative connotations. The term should therefore be avoided.[97] In general, terminological caution is required: "The use of the term 'cloning' by the media when describing this technique has unfortunate connotations conjuring up as it does images of

---

88 HGAC/HFEA, *Cloning Issues*, 9.3., 33.
89 Ibid., Summary, 3.
90 Department of Health (DoH), *CMO Report*, ES 1, 5.
91 DoH, *Stem Cell Research: Medical Progress with Responsibility. A Report from the Chief Medical Officer's Expert Group Reviewing the Potential of Developments in Stem Cell Research and Cell Nuclear Replacement to Benefit Human Health* (June 2000).
92 DoH, *CMO Report*, 2, 16.
93 Ibid., 3, 32.
94 Ibid., 4, 37.
95 Ibid., chapter 2.
96 Ibid., 1.8, 13.
97 Ibid., 1.15, 15.

whole people or parts of people being created or of babies being created as a source of spare parts."[98] In order to avoid the term *cloning* in the context of medical research the CMO report describes the "technical procedures"[99] and suggests (in accordance with the HGAC/HFEA Report) the term "cell nuclear replacement techniques" (CNR). These techniques are used, it explains, "to create embryos up to a maximum of 14 days old for research."[100]

The CMO's Expert Group emphasises that embryonic stem cell research is basic medical research which at the moment "would precede, probably by many years, any possible application to treatment."[101] The successful application of research still depends upon

"Whether stem cells can be successfully isolated and grown in the laboratory; whether stem cells grown in the laboratory can be influenced to turn into specific cell types; whether stem cells that have formed particular cell types could be used to treat patients whose tissue was diseased or damaged through injury; whether tissue grown in this way would develop normally or whether there might be risks to the patient."[102]

Yet despite these caveats, the benefits for a "wide range" of people's health are considered to be "significant",[103] "substantial",[104] "enormous",[105] and "great".[106]

The expert advisory group accepts the fourteen days limit for embryo research first proposed by the Warnock Report.[107] The group is adamant that the position of special status does not imply any consequentialist type of morality; the human embryo, independent of an action's consequences, deserves "a measure of respect"[108] beyond that accorded to embryos of other species. It is accorded this measure of respect due to its biologically human characteristics and because of its potential for full human existence.[109] The respect owed increases as it develops, the report says. Once the embryo has reached fourteen days of development and beyond, its respect is absolute *at least in the context of research*. Until then, its value can be weighed against the potential therapeutic benefits arising from the proposed research.[110] The CMO Report reaches the conclusion that

"The current restrictions and controls on embryo research reflect this [...] view, providing the human embryo with a degree of protection in law but allowing the benefits of the proposed research to be weighed against the respect to the embryo."[111]

---

98   DoH, *CMO Report*, 4.15, 40.
99   Ibid., 1.15, 15.
100 Ibid.
101 Ibid., ES 2, 5.
102 Ibid., ES 3, 5.
103 Ibid., ES 18, 8.
104 Ibid., ES 20, 8.
105 Ibid., ES 24, 9.
106 Ibid., ES 25, 9.
107 Ibid., 4.12, 39.
108 Ibid., 4.10, 39.
109 Ibid., ES 17, 7.
110 Ibid., 39.
111 Ibid., ES 17, 7.

Against the background of possible health benefits the Report endorses the extension of research purposes in the 1990 Act, the permission to clone human embryos for research[112] and the destruction of human embryos prior to fourteen days of development which such research includes. The greater the potential benefit of the research and the wider the range of people that can benefit from it, the more respectful and ethically justified such research may be, the Report concludes.[113]

The moral weight of therapeutic benefits is seen as increasing in accordance with the number of people that can benefit from such therapies. As the reports state, the greater the amount of people able to share in the benefits of a particular avenue of research, the more morally worthy such research becomes. The number of people benefiting from certain research seems to work as a factor x which increases the research's moral weight allowing it to outweigh other morally weighty ends.

The documents appear less concerned with what it means to be *a* healthy human being, and more with how to achieve a healthy population, healthy human *beings*. The particular patient exists as part of a group of people "constructed as desperate and requiring intervention at the level of politics on behalf of science and medicine."[114] Diseases, health, and research with therapeutic aims concern *collectives of sufferers*. What matters are "the patients suffering from a wide range of incurable disorders."[115] What is weighed up against the value of early embryonic life is "the health of the population."[116] The HoL Select Committee Report points at the distinction when recommending a discussion of the term *serious disease* where it states "it is uncertain whether it means serious for the individual or serious for society."[117] The concern of public health policy making is with the "many Britons [who have] spent years of their lives carrying the burden of chronic disease rather than enjoying healthy years of life."[118] The focus on sufferers (plural) rather than the particular person (singular) seems to represent a framing of the arguments according to the responsibilities of the parliamentary system, namely to consider the population (the electorate) and economic factors.[119]

112 DoH, *CMO Report*, Recommendations 1 and 4, 45–46.
113 Ibid., 4.10, 39.
114 Parry, "Politics of Cloning", 159.
115 DoH, *CMO Report*, 1.7, 13.
116 Ibid., 2.1, 16.
117 HoL, Report, 8.8, 39.
118 DoH, *CMO Report*, 2.1, 16.
119 Cf. Parry, "Politics of Cloning", 155–159. We might still ask ourselves if sense be made of such a *quantitative factor* in the (qualitative) evaluation of ends and actions. And more particularly, can sense be made of it where what is at the other end of the balancing scales is a personal human life – even where it exists perhaps as a possibility only? Where the prohibition of killing is taken seriously as placing human life *categorically* (i.e. a difference in kind, not degree) outside the value scales of positive goods such as health, no matter how great the quantitative factor x might be, it can never tip the scales against life and in favour of health. Whilst the positive good of health can increase in weight if many healthy people are added up, it can still not outweigh the prohibition of killing, which as a negative prohibition points to

The UK Government in its response of August 2000 accepted the Report's recommendations in full.[120] Draft regulations were brought to Parliament, debated and passed by the House of Commons on 19 December 2000 and by the House of Lords on 22 January 2001. Three new purposes were added to the five in the 1990 Act. Additional licences for research on embryos can be issued where such research seeks (a) to increase knowledge about the development of the embryo, (b) to increase knowledge about serious disease, or (c) enable any such knowledge to be applied in developing treatments for serious disease.

2.2.4 The 2002 HoL Select Committee Report

As a result of the debates on the regulations and the attempts to apply for leave, the House of Lords (HoL) established a Select Committee. Its remit was to consider the issues connected with human cloning and stem cell research and to review the justification of the regulations.[121] The results of the review are largely in line with the previous two reports and were published in 2002.[122]

After introducing the background of the Committee's inquiry in chapter one, the Committee's Report looks into the potential of both embryonic and adult stem cells (chapters two and three), discusses the status of the early embryo (chapter four), the techniques involved in cloning and embryonic stem cell research (chapter five), commercial interests[123] (chapter six), and finally legislation and regulation, including an international dimension (chapters seven and eight).

It recognises the great therapeutic potential of human embryonic stem cells and views that as basis for "a strong scientific and medical case for continued research on human ES cells."[124] The Report speaks about "cell-based treatments, both to repair or replace tissues damaged by fractures, burns and other injuries and to treat a wide range of very common degenerative diseases, such as Alzheimer's disease, cardiac failure, diabetes, and Parkinson's disease."[125] It strongly recommends the fourteen days limit as proposed by Mary Warnock's Committee.[126]

---

life's categorically different value status, which will be discussed more fully as part of the following reflection on health.

120 *Government Response to the Recommendations Made in the Chief Medical Officer's Expert Group Report "Stem Cell Research: Medical Progress with Responsibility"* (August 2000), Foreword, 1.

121 HoL, *Report*, 5.

122 HoL, *Stem Cell Research. Report from the Select Committee* (13.02.2002).

123 The HoL Committee is alone in addressing commercial interests though it admits to doing so in a very limited fashion. "Since we have received only a limited amount of evidence on this aspect of the subject and were unable to probe further within our time constraint, we simply identify the issues which have come to our attention. They are, however, of considerable significance for the legal and regulatory control of stem cell research, in which companies involved in stem cell research have an obvious interest." (HoL, *Report*, 6.1., 32).

124 HoL, *Report*, Conclusion vi, 48.

125 HoL, *Report*, 2.6, 11. (my italics).

126 Ibid., Conclusion vii, 48.

Whilst it agrees with an extension of the research purposes, it invites the Department of Health (DoH) to draw up guidance on the definition of "serious disease" in order to avoid uncertainty.[127] And it concludes that

> "At an appropriate time, perhaps towards the end of the decade, the Government should undertake a further review of scientific progress of adult stem cell research and therapies, and of the development of stem cell banks, with a view to determining whether research on human embryos is still necessary."[128]

In support of the fourteen-day-mark the HoL select committee states that a qualitative leap would mark the process of development of the embryo, which otherwise is a "continual process of change."[129] Only for the sake of convenience, the select committee's Report says, is this continual process commonly described in terms of stages. Yet the process nevertheless involves at least one distinct change. In the first two weeks post-fertilisation the cells of the embryo are "still relatively undifferentiated and there is no trace of human structure such as a nervous system, and hence there can be no sentience."[130] Leaving aside the biologically questionable statement that "a nervous system" or "sentience" is in any way distinctively human, the appearance of the primitive streak is affirmed as the line beyond which one should not move.

Some ascribe full rights and respect even to the embryo prior to fourteen days, the HoL Report says, for it has not been demonstrated yet that the early embryo is not a person. "They suggest that early embryos should therefore be given the 'benefit of the doubt': even if they are not persons they should be treated as if they were persons, and accorded the full rights that were accorded to persons."[131] But, the HoL committee revealingly counters, if there are morally weighty reasons for doing research on embryos (that is, the relief of suffering caused by disease)[132] a decision must be reached "on the basis of arguments that fall short of proof."[133]

As for the health benefits of stem cells generally and embryonic stem cells in particular, none of the scientific witnesses to the HoL Select Committee "seriously questioned the therapeutic potential of stem cells for a wide range of disorders"[134] so that the advance of knowledge possibly beneficial for clinical medi-

---

127 HoL, *Report*, 11, 47.

128 Ibid., Conclusion xix, 49–50.

129 Ibid., 4.2, 20. Nobel Prize winning biologist Christine Nüsslein-Vollhardt argues that biologically nothing is more *discontinuous* than a process which, at nidation, requires direct cellular contact with another organism and which, at birth, ends in a separate, independent organism (Nüsslein-Vollhardt, *Von Genen und Embryonen*, 68).

130 HoL, *Report*, 4.2 (d), 20.

131 Ibid., 4.15, 22. As we will see later, this is the position that would recommend itself on the basis of an Augustinian anthropology.

132 Ibid., 4.17, 22.

133 Ibid., 4.16, 22. Against the idea that a decision must be reached on the basis of arguments that fall short of proof see Robert Song, 'To Be Willing to Kill What for All One Knows Is A Person Is to Be Willing to Kill a Person', in: Waters/Cole-Turner: *God and the Embryo: Religious Voices on Stem Cells and Cloning* (Washington, 2003), 98–107.

134 HoL, *Report*, 2.10, 12.

cine was a strong enough argument to be weighed against the special value and respect granted the embryo.[135]

2.2.5 Concluding remarks

In all three documents, the intrinsic worth of the pursuit of health answered positively the question of whether or not human embryos should be used in research. The value of the pre-fourteen day embryo was weighed up against the value of potential health of (born) humans. Human embryonic stem cell research (and the use of human embryos "at a very early stage")[136] was considered morally worthy and legally permissible as long as it showed the potential of benefiting the health of human beings.

The documents considered the embryo prior to fourteen days as *not yet a full human being* with the potential of *becoming* a full human being. Therefore, it should be accorded a measure of respect. Human life demands respect; not fully realised human life demands at least a measure of respect. The embryo's value increases up to a point of its development, fourteen days in the reports. After this point its value is too great to be outweighed by the value of potential health benefits; after this point the reports recommend the prohibition of the destruction of embryos for research purposes *however great the potential of health might be.*

However, and this is an important *addendum*, even after fourteen days of development, the embryo's value is still not absolute according to current legislation. Its life can be taken away without it being considered the unlawful killing of another human being. Depending on national abortion legislation the termination of life is sometimes allowed for the whole gestation period up until the moment of birth, for instance in the case of severe genetic disorders and/or disabilities. Here late terminations are not uncommon. Only after birth is the value absolute in that it would be considered infanticide to take away a newborn's life in case of severe physical impairments.

Research for health benefits is considered a great good – yet it is not a great enough good to justify the use of embryos at later developmental stages. At later gestation stages never the health benefits for others but only the *potential risks to the embryo's own or its mother's health and life* can justify the termination of its life. After fourteen days of development, the embryo seems to count as a human subject covered by the moral code of medical research and practice as enshrined in the 1964 *Declaration of Helsinki*.[137]

The 1998–2002 policy documents, however, did not explicitly reflect on human life, human relationships, and the meaning of health. Whilst advancing health as main reason for research, what it means to be "a healthy human being" is a

---

135 DoH, *CMO Report*, ES 17, 7.
136 HoL, *Report*, 4.11, 39.
137 Declaration of Helsinki: http://bmj.bmjjournals.com/cgi/content/full/313/7070/1448/a, last accessed 04/2010.

question that remains unasked and unexplored. Taking into account the practical, political, and moral implications of the end of health that trumps other values, the absence of philosophical exploration is critical indeed.

3. CONCEPTUALISING HEALTH (1): EARLY PHILOSOPHICAL AND THEOLOGICAL REFLECTIONS

Since the beginnings of Western medicine the concept of health and practices of healing were subject to debates and reflections. The chapter before us turns to such discussion. I will engage with the doctor-philosopher Galen of Pergamon, who lived and worked in the second century AD in the Roman Empire. His "dominion over medicine"[138] lasted at least until the Renaissance. In a second step, I will engage with theologians of the early Church and their analysis of natural medicine of Galen's provenance.

Galen developed an idea of health as the normal, that is natural, state of the body. Yet Galen moves beyond a purely naturalist or individualised welfare account of health and of medical practice. He emphasises the union of body and soul, and the corrective influence of reason or the rational soul on human behaviour.

This allows humans to recognise *general* principles for the improvement both of the constitution of the body and the affections of the soul. The recognition of the union of body and soul on the one hand, and of generally recognisable rational principles on the other allows him to develop an account of medical epistemology and practice which is both general and individualised, and on which a common medical morality may be built.

The following analysis of Galen's views is guided by questions, which point to his Christian contemporaries and to his philosophical successors. What, according to Galen, is human life (that is, the life of the patient)? How does he understand the natural (that is, the body)? What is the personal (in Galen's terms, the soul) and what is its relation to the body? In what state of being is the patient when he or she approaches the doctor (what is disease according to Galen)? What state of being does the patient wish for (what is health for Galen)? Finally, what methods does the doctor use to answer these questions? And what epistemological method does Galen suggest for the doctor?

Most of Galen's Christian contemporaries did not share his optimism regarding medicine's promises. This came with a view that medical knowledge and philosophical reflection *alone* were insufficient for achieving true well-being or fullness of life. This is not to say that they rejected medicine as a means of restoring health. And it is also not to say that a uniform body of opinion existed in the Church of the first centuries. It was scarcely a monolithic community. It existed in three geographical spheres, each with their own language (Greek, Latin, and Syrian), each rooted within their particular cultural and philosophical traditions, and each with their distinct theological schools. In the Greek-speaking East theologians such as Origen, Basil the Great, Gregory of Nyssa, and Gregory of

138 Porter, *Greatest Benefit to Mankind*, 73.

Nazianzus viewed Christ as the teacher who leads humans to the good or full life. For theologians in the Latin-speaking West, humans needed to be healed, renewed or transformed by Christ (often called "the physician") before being able to perform good and meaningful action.[139] In contrast to the Western and Eastern Church, the Syrian Church, the smallest and most diverse of all three, focused less on Christological creeds and more on hymns and liturgy as a form of praise of God's magnitude as revealed in the incarnation of Christ.[140]

The differences in Christology and emphasis on action and liturgy were accompanied by a differing appreciation of nature, naturalist medicine and the philosophy that accompanied it. Referring to the New Testament stories of healing, the majority of early Church theologians shared an appreciation of bodily health and healing.

Against historians of medicine, such as Vivian Nutton, who described the early Christian focus on healing as in competition with medicine, nineteenth century German theologian Adolf von Harnack defended the primacy of salvation over bodily health whilst at the same time establishing his thesis of Christianity as a medical religion.

In "Medicinisches aus Ältester Kirchengeschichte"[141] von Harnack looks at the relationship of ancient medicine and early Christianity, and the ways in which the example of Jesus Christ and his apostles influenced medical practice of the first centuries. He explores *historically* the relationship between Christianity and a medicine that is based on the knowledge of natural processes and the principles of logical analysis, experience, hypothesis and testing through experiments. Yet any compilation of historical material, he concedes, is only moved beyond the accidental if viewed in the context of the New Testament's gospel of Jesus Christ who promised and brought healing for humanity.[142] The relationship between medicine and Christianity needs to be viewed *theologically* in light of the New Testament's message of salvation, which locates medicine within the order of salvation.

Against the background of the thematic prevalence of healing in the New Testament and the historical context of early Church approaches to medicine as collected by von Harnack, this chapter analyses three early Christians' views of disease, health, and medical healing.

I will look at Tatian, a second century Syrian theologian and outspoken critic of naturalist medicine, Tertullian, a contemporary of Tatian's from the Latin-speaking Western Church, and Basil the Great, fourth century bishop and theologian of the Greek-speaking Eastern Church, who defended naturalist medicine as serving human progress towards greater union with God. The analysis will include

---

139 This emphasis on action still persists in the Western Christian tradition where the focus is on how one *acts* as the measure of faith. In the Eastern tradition (and this will be apparent, too, in the Church Fathers treated here) the *liturgy*, the act of worship in community, is the source and measure and life-giver to all other parts of life in faith.

140 Geerlings, *Theologen*, 12.

141 "Medical ideas in the history of the early Church" (here and in the following translations are my own).

142 Harnack, Medicinisches aus Ältester Kirchengeschichte, 125.

the Cappadocian Fathers Gregory of Nazianzus and Gregory of Nyssa, who described Basil's attitude towards medicine, as well as Origen, who is a central reference point of Basil's account of medicine. However, Greek writer John Chrysostom, who showed an interest in medical tools and therapeutic applications, will not be treated here. As his concern was with practical details of treatment such as surgical instruments or pharmacological drugs, his writings are of primarily historical interest.

Choosing these writers allows me to engage with the three theological traditions characteristic of the early Church, Western and Eastern Christian traditions. Above all, it allows me to capture and explore the broad range of attitudes towards naturalist medicine found across the early Church.

Tatian, Tertullian, and Basil take as a starting point the body-soul union lodged within humanity's union with God. They do not conceptualise this union functionally like Galen, but hierarchically and metaphysically, that is, in the soul's transcending the body in orientation to Christ.

Whilst there is some agreement in the area of anthropology in its orientation to Christ,[143] the three writers reach different conclusions as to the need for, and usefulness of, medicine. Such disagreement stems from a difference in opinion as to the relationship between the natural, demons and the divine as played out in the body. Such interplay is foundational for the writers' views on disease and leads to a greater or lesser degree of scepticism towards medicine's capacity of bringing about health and well-being.

Tatian saw the human body as good where it is in union with the soul and the divine (or holy) spirit. However, after the Fall, this union is severely disrupted and under constant threat. The body is vulnerable to the attack and entry of demons. Diseases of the body are caused by demons, evil forces *in* nature acting *upon* nature. Healing of the body can be achieved *not* through naturalist medicine (for it is in nature that demons dwell) but through the power of God's word. Tatian's demonology as explicated in the *Oratio ad Graecos*, one of his few remaining works, led to his sharp rejection of naturalist pharmacological knowledge. He was denounced a heretic by the Church due to his proximity to the Gnostic movement.[144] However, Tatian's overall concern was *not* to attack medicine or one of its branches but to enable true human-ness and human flourishing.

Second century Church theologian Tertullian draws a distinction between physical and spiritual sickness. Spiritual sickness is caused by heretical belief and requires the divine cure of the word. Physical diseases can be caused by natural entities inflicting the body but also by demons. Whilst the former requires the doctor's knowledge of natural processes, demons need to be exorcised through the power of God's word. Tertullian's treatment of the sacrament of baptism underlines his *hierarchical* view of the body-soul union. Spiritual health and healing is valued higher than physical health and medical cures. It alone can lead to eternal flourishing and true human fulfilment, which is Tertullian's overall concern.

---

143 Cf. Frings, *Medizin und Arzt bei Kirchenvätern*, B.6.
144 Cramer, *Geist Gottes in frühsyrischer Theologie*, 47–48.

Medicine does not need to be rejected – it is not demonic – yet its importance is limited by the greater good of spiritual healing performed by Jesus Christ and his successors in the sacraments of the Church.

Unlike both Tertullian and Tatian, Basil the Great saw diseases as having their cause in nature. He rejects the idea of interplay between nature and evil spirits. This allowed him to support medical knowledge and practice, which he saw as an art given to humanity by God so that it may enable health and human flourishing. Medicine reflects God's will for human salvation, Basil says. Humans should call in the doctor but not leave off hoping in God. Jesus' example leads Basil to reflect on medical practice in the context of the good life. He comes to view medicine as an act of *charity* in that it is meant to involve not only *curing* but also *caring* for the sick. This conclusion has had implications for medical practice also beyond Basil's life times.

Whilst Basil developed his view of medical care from the gospel narratives, in particular the care shown by Jesus and his apostles to the sick and underprivileged, he nowhere explicates the theological anthropology that underlies such care. Neither do the other writers in their contexts. This is, then, the main weakness of their reflection on the meaning of health for it leads to a failure of recognising implications on the personal level of existence. Against this background, I explore Augustine's fully coherent theological understanding of human life in chapter four. The distinction of physical and spiritual sickness to which Tatian, Tertullian and Basil point and which legitimises and limits the art and science of medicine is a lead that is worth exploring in more detail: it, too, will be taken up in the context of St Augustine's work.

3.1 HEALTH, WELL-BEING, AND THE ROLE OF REASON: GALEN OF PERGAMON

In his day, Galen of Pergamon was widely recognised as an anatomist, physician, philosopher of medicine, and writer. Today's historians of medicine consider him the endpoint of some seven hundred years of consolidation of Greek and Roman medicine. His work is acknowledged as the repository of a number of ideas on which modern medicine has been built. Drawing on the philosophy of Plato and Aristotle as well as the Hippocratic School, Galen was the first in the history of Western medicine to articulate the importance of both hypotheses and experience for medical knowledge and practice.[145]

In spite of the loss of about one-third of his treatises, more than 120 authentic titles have survived[146] though some only in their Arabic translation. In the following, I draw on *The Art of Medicine, On the Therapeutic Method, To Thrasyboulos*

---

145 Porter, *Greatest Benefit to Mankind*, 82. For an account of Galen's life and formative years see Hankinson, *Galen on Therapeutic Method*, ix–xxxiv/Nutton, "Method of Healing", 1–25/Nutton, *Early Career*, 158–171/Siegel, *Galen's System of Physiology*, 4–26.
146 Siegel, *Galen's System of Physiology*, 1.

on the question *Is Healthiness a Part of Medicine or Gymnastics* and *The Best Doctor is also a Philosopher* as well as Galen's work on body and soul such as *The Affections and Errors of the Soul*, *The Soul's Dependence on the Body*, and *The Best Constitution of our Bodies*.

Galen's recognition of bodily reality allows him to defend a shared body of medical knowledge, to which he made contributions of the highest order with his own (mainly anatomical) research. His recognition of the individual (though not autonomous) character allowed him to reflect on moral agency more generally and the moral conduct of doctors in particular. Due to his emphasis on rational, philosophical training he was able to defend a code of professional conduct which eliminates vices and enhances virtues, thus enabling the doctor to work towards the patient's health rather than his own wealth.

3.1.1 Logic and medical epistemology

Though originally earmarked for a career in philosophy, when Galen was sixteen or seventeen the decision was taken that he should devote himself to medicine. Philosophy, however, remained a subject of great importance. It should promote medicine, Galen taught, and a physician should devote himself to philosophical analysis and enquiry.

Galen did not belong to one particular philosophical or medical school. His principal philosophical debt was to the schools of Plato and Aristotle; his medical debt to Hippocrates who had lived and worked about 550 years earlier. He imagined a unified philosophico-medical tradition, beginning with Hippocrates through to Plato and Aristotle and then to himself.[147]

Galen recognised and promoted Hippocrates as both an outstanding practitioner and medical theorist, and one analytically superior to the medical schools that continued to exist until the second century AD. He declared Hippocrates the intellectual father of a new medicine based on reason, experience, and observation. He identified him as the originator of the physical and physiological theory of the four primary qualities and the four elements of the world on which Galen himself was to build his own medical system. Galen accepted ideas of other medical sects[148] only as long as they were compatible with what he understood to be the Hippocratic method. He proposed that a hypothesis, suggested by chance, inspiration or analogous reasoning might be tested against, and justified through, experience. He thought the Dogmatist sect was right to stress the necessity of analogies,

---

147 Barnes, "Galen on Logic and Therapy", 51.
148 *Hippocratic Writings*, *Tradition in Medicine*, 79. Dogmatists defended against the Empiricists a medicine based on hypotheses and *analogous reasoning*. In order to arrive at knowledge of the underlying structure of the body and the nature of its pathological condition, the doctor needed to infer from apparent signs to the hidden, internal conditions of the patient's body. Empiricists, by contrast, proceeded by building up general statements of connections between observable items and accused Dogmatists of reducing the medical art to a simple matter of postulates.

inferring from visible symptoms an understanding of the hidden causes or inquiring as to the relation of form and function in anatomy and physiology. Yet for him analogous reasoning needed to be "intimately connected with empirical knowledge and observation: the securest kind of knowledge [...] is that based on sound anatomical research in conjunction with a syllogistic presentation of the argument."[149] Galen's eclectic and synthetic method ultimately led to the disappearance of the competing medical sects of his times or, rather, to their survival in his own medical theory.[150]

A striking fact about Galen's medical epistemology is the importance he ascribes to logic. Exact medical knowledge of the human body is the result of logical thought.[151] Without logic, a physician's diagnostic, prognostic and therapeutic success is random.[152] Yet it is never logical reasoning *in abstracto* but reasoning that takes place in practice at a particular patient's bedside. That is, it is always bound up with, and shaped by, not only the requirements of the patient's specific body but moreover and essentially so by the doctor's view of the patient's life as well as the understanding he has of the moral duties of the medical profession (*vide infra*). Galen himself took pride in being both what one would call today a moral philosopher, a clinician and a medical scientist.

3.1.2 Functional view of body and soul

Galen was at the patient's bedside, studied anatomy, pathology and physiology (the main fields of medicine in the second century), performed dissections and conducted live experiments on animals. Galen's anthropology is derived from such experimental research, which he combined with astute philosophical and logical enquiry. It is essentially *functional*.

Humans need the various parts of their bodies not for what they are, but for what they do, Galen says. A body's purpose is its *activities* or *functions*. Humans need organs only for the sake of their activities: "What we actually need is to see, hear, talk, and walk, as opposed to eyes, ears, tongue or legs."[153] In this sense, not any unnatural condition of the body should be called disease, but only those that have a perceptible, damaging effect on bodily functions. Galen insists that diseases properly so-called must be more than simply out-of-the-ordinary conditions of the body. They must involve damage to at least one of its characteristic activities. Only organ conditions that affect the overall *organ activity* require medical therapy.[154]

---

149 Singer, *Galen*, xv.
150 Ibid.
151 Galen, *The Order of My Own Books*, 24. Cf. also Siegel, *Galen's System of Physiology*, 16.
152 Galen, *The Order of My Own Books*, 23–25; *The Best Doctor is Also a Philosopher*, 30/33-
       34. Cf. Barnes, "Galen on Logic and Therapy", 52/65 ff.
153 Galen, *Therapeutic Method*, I.9.3.
154 Ibid.

Galen is interested in bodily reality in terms of its functions, not its material properties. However, it needs to be noted in this context that *matter* in Galen's thought does not correspond to what one understands today by the term, as Singer points out: "Material substances in ancient thought – e.g. earth, fire, pneuma – each tend to be endowed with their individual properties, in a way which distinguishes them from the 'fundamental particles' of our reductionist system."[155]

Galen's interpretation of teleology and functionality has its philosophical origin in Plato[156] but above all in Aristotle.[157] Particular activities are a particular organ's purpose or *telos*, the end or final cause of the organ's structures being arranged the way they are. For Aristotle, all purposeful development in nature must take place according to a first cause which is the unmoved moving force. Aristotle avoided metaphysical or religious expressions that would indicate the action of a personalised god such as it is found in the Hebrew-Christian tradition. This being the case, *demiourgos* or *the unmoved moving force* for Aristotle is a formative principle in nature. Galen seemed to have used the term similarly: he spoke of the demiurge as biological phenomenon, and an objective, depersonalised force or mind that occupies the space around us. His interpretation of teleology in nature appears impersonal, and rational.[158]

The soul, for Galen, is real, too: it belongs to natural reality. Galen's ideas about the soul do not represent a precise, uniform and consistent system.[159] The physician need not speculate about the nature of the human soul; all he needs to know, Galen says, is that the soul refers to a certain set of bodily functions which are located primarily in three organs. The functions unite body and soul; they are in union *via* their functions.

Galen saw the soul not as an independent substance or even agent but as of one composition with the body.[160] Being of humoral composition like the body, the soul is temporal and belongs to the sphere of temporal nature, of *physics* not *metaphysics*. Soul and body are no material opposites; the soul is also understood in terms of its functions. It refers to a group of distinct bodily functions such as brain functions, sleep, memory or imagination, and also emotions and desires. These functions can be located in the three organs of brain, heart and liver, which were therefore considered the seat of the soul.[161] In this sense, Galen's functional understanding of the human body and its organs extends itself to his view of the soul.

Whilst Aristotle's influence on Galen's understanding of the soul seems beyond question,[162] according to Siegel[163] Galen's agreement went no further than to

155 Singer, *Galen*, xxxii.
156 Plato, *Republic*, 357b–358a.
157 Aristotle, *Metaphysics*, 1013 a 15/Aristotle, *Nicomachean Ethics*, I.7.
158 Siegel, *Galen and Nervous System*, 13.
159 Ibid., 114.
160 Ibid., 18.
161 Galen, *Soul's Dependence on the Body*, 157.
162 See for instance Galen's recognition of Aristotle (and also Plato) in *The Soul's Dependence on the Body*, 160–164.

say that the soul is nothing more than the functional (formal and vital) principle of the body's actions. He did not approve of Aristotle's idea of the rational soul, the highest or ruling part of the soul, as something divine that entered the body from the outside. Reason, for Galen, originates in material processes such as the mixture of humours which determine the composition of the brain. Reason then is perishable like all material processes and activities.[164] The soul does not and cannot outlast the life of the body.[165]

3.1.3 Health as metabolic balance

Against the background of Galen's functional view of human life both in body and soul, how did he view the patient's state of health? The natural condition, Galen says, is to function; the unnatural condition is the total failure or the impairment of function.[166] Health, then, is the natural condition and is the ability to function; disease is not to function.

> "Who does not understand that if hearing is health, then impairment of hearing and deafness will be illnesses? Similarly, if digestion is healthy, then bad digestion or the complete lack of it are illnesses; and if voluntary movement is healthy, then spasm, palpitation, paralysis, tremor, in short anything that either completely destroys voluntary motion or else interferes with it in some way, is an illness."[167]

Health or the natural condition, the balance of qualities or the functioning of organs, Galen says, is that which humanity strives for; disease is that which humans try to avoid.

> "Surely everyone would agree in not wanting any part unable to perform its function – eyes unable to see, for example, a nose unable to smell, legs unable to walk, or in general, any part which either does not perform its function at all or performs it badly."[168]

Humans desire the removal of obstacles to these activities; they desire the removal of illness.[169] In accordance with his teleological view of nature, Galen explains that physicians should use their art, the "understanding of things healthy and morbid"[170] to restore the natural functions of the body.

> "The first and most particular concern of doctors, indeed the thing which is pretty well the defining feature of their business, is the removal of illnesses. For as soon as this is accomplished, the damage to the activity disappears, and all the other symptoms are removed along with it."[171]

---

163 Siegel, *Galen and Nervous System*, 119.
164 Ibid., 130.
165 Galen, *Soul's Dependence on the Body*, 152–153.
166 Galen, *To Thrasyboulos*, 61.
167 Galen, *Therapeutic Method*, I.7.15.
168 Galen, *To Thrasyboulos*, 61.
169 Galen, *Therapeutic Method*, II.3.10.
170 Galen, *To Thrasyboulos*, 58.
171 Galen, *Therapeutic Method*, II.3.10.

Health and illness belong to the same genus, namely the body and its parts and organs. They are first of all states of the human body.[172] In *The Art of Medicine*, Galen defined health as the "good *mixture* of the simple, primary parts, and good *proportion* in the organs which are composed of these."[173] Here, Galen's language refers back to the teachings of both Plato and the Hippocratic School:[174] a common core of Plato's concept of health is to "look upon health as a kind of harmony, balance, and order."[175] Disease is a lack of balance; it is disproportion and disorder.

Galen defined the principle of metabolic transformation within the body as the constant transfer, interchange and exchange of qualities such as hot, cold, dry, moist, dense, viscous or hard, thus affecting the balance of qualities within the parts of the body and within the bodily humours (blood, phlegm, yellow bile and black bile)[176] with an increased likeliness of a lack of balance, and hence, disease. The humours were also related to the four seasons (blood to summer and spring, phlegm to winter, yellow bile to summer and fall, black bile to autumn):[177] the seasons were thought to affect the balance of the qualities and of the bodily parts, organs and humours. Medicine's task is to restore impaired bodily functions by way of restoration of humoral balance.

> "Some overseer is required to take care of them, to recognise what substance a body is lacking, and how much of this substance, and to cure the loss immediately by introducing the same amount of substance."[178]

Whilst using terms such as *normal* in the context of health definitions, Galen nowhere sought to define *quantitatively* what he called "normal equilibrium". In *The Pulse for Beginners*, he gives an idea of the *qualitative* factors that might disturb the equilibrium, such as the climate, hot or cold bathing, or type, quantity and frequency of meals.[179] It can only be inferred that in accordance with Plato[180] *the natural* (which is *the normal*) is the intermediate position between (too much) warmth and (too much) cold, or (too much) wet and (too much) dry.

On the one hand, the natural condition of the organism indicates for Galen the result of generation and growth. On the other hand, it is not only a static, but also a kinetic concept: the elements of the organism function according to their specific purpose which forms part of the general *purpose and goal* of the bodily organism and natural existence.[181] Galen's talk of the natural condition, hence of health and disease, has its place in a *teleological view* of nature.

---

172 Galen, *To Thrasyboulos*, 55–59.
173 Galen, *The Art of Medicine*, 347. My italics.
174 Hippocrates, *The Nature of Man*, 4.
175 Petersson, "Health in Plato's Thought", 3.
176 Hippocrates, *The Nature of Man*, 4 ff.
177 Siegel, *Galen's System of Physiology*, 217. Cf. Hippocrates, *Airs-Waters-Places*, 2/11.
178 Galen, *To Thrasyboulos*, 69.
179 Galen, *The Pulses for Beginners*, 332–333.
180 Petersson, "Health in Plato's Thought", 8.
181 Siegel, *Galen and Nervous System*, 10.

3.1.4 Concluding remarks

Galen's unequivocal recognition of the reality of the body can be foundational for generally recognisable disease definitions, hence, for a shared body of medical knowledge. The question remains whether the anthropological and epistemological framework that Galen develops allows for a widely shared understanding of professional duties. Can there be any form of *moral agency* where the soul is understood to be functional, dependent upon bodily functions and of humoral composition as the body? Galen's *functional union* of body and soul as looked at so far is not sufficient to answer this question.

Yet Galen's understanding of the soul goes beyond its dependence upon the body. In *The Affections and Errors of the Soul* he distinguishes irrational and rational functions of the soul, and involuntary and voluntary human acts. The source of involuntary acts is a person's irrational soul or particular character, "qualities [...] endowed by Nature."[182] A person's *character* is biologically determined: every individual is born with his or her distinctive character, which depends on the distinct mixture of qualities.[183] This mixture differs from individual to individual. Thus a person's *character* is independent of upbringing or education, as examples of young children show.[184] Emotions or "affections" in Galen's terminology such as anger or shame, Galen says, are irrational affections that result from a change of proportion in the mixture of qualities that make up a person's character. They arise from "irrational impulse."[185] As with diseases, climate, bathing, type, quantity and frequency of meals influence this mixture, and hence, make us more passionate, angry, furious or more level headed, calm, collected.[186]

Now, involuntary acts and character can be and should be improved under the influence of voluntary acts rooted in human *reason*. As Galen remarks, even at the age of fifty one should not put aside the possibility of improving the soul voluntarily – for if one's body was in a bad stage at this age, one would not give oneself up to bad condition.[187] Nature, Galen says, "is the major factor in achieving a good life in childhood, but later [...] the major factors are doctrine and practice"[188] and our susceptibility to rational, philosophical training.

Did Galen not understand reason in terms of humoral mixtures, too? Is reason not biological, too? Indeed, he viewed reason as being dependent on the mixture of the humours and the composition of the brain.[189] Yet notwithstanding this, he conceived of the soul's rational aspect as being independent of human biology – at least in a sense. Reason originates in a mixture of elements in the brain (thus depends upon physiology) *yet at the same time* it is a function open to philosophi-

---

182 Galen, *Affections and Errors of the Soul*, 119.
183 Galen, *Soul's Dependence on the Body*, 167.
184 Galen, *Affections and Errors of the Soul*, 117.
185 Ibid., 103.
186 Galen, *Soul's Dependence on the Body*, 150; 158–159.
187 Galen, *Affections and Errors of the Soul*, 106.
188 Ibid., 117.
189 Galen, *Soul's Dependence on the Body*, 167–168.

cal thoughts and ideas, thus to *philosophical training*. Education and training shape the rational aspect of the soul, which in this *is independent of biological influences*. As such, it may influence the irrational, biological aspects of the soul – the character humans are born with, their emotional afflictions. "Training and education dispel evil, and engender good."[190]

Galen confronted the alternative of either allowing the somatic condition to determine passions, emotions *and* rational thought completely or of understanding reason as a power that may rule and modify the physical condition by modifying the "affections and errors of the soul". Where humans lack philosophical training *in combination* with specific somatic imbalances, morally bad actions may result. Where they receive philosophical training, their soul's irrational aspects can be corrected. Reason modifies human traits of character.[191] "Those […] who are in the grip of moderate affections […] will be able to make their soul free and noble by the ministrations of reason."[192]

Now, to return to the question of a code of professional morality: Galen was painfully aware that such a code was needed for the medical profession. Otherwise, doctors would be essentially "on the make", he said. He challenged his contemporaries, in particular their uncontrolled greed, interrogating whether there was any single one

> "Of whom it may be said that his desire for financial gain is limited to what will provide for his simple bodily needs? Is there one with the ability not only to make a verbal formulation, but also to give an actual example of this: The limitation of wealth to Nature's requirements for the prevention of hunger, thirst, or cold?"[193]

In this context, Galen advocated philosophical training so as to improve the doctors' greedy character. Vices in a doctor can be painfully dangerous for the patient, Galen points out: a doctor called Socles, who "promising to set Diodorus back straight, piled three solid stones, each four feet square, on the hunch-back's spine. Diodorus was crushed and died, but he became straighter than a rule."[194] Where, in contrast, a doctor is equipped with philosophical knowledge and an understanding of the moral life in terms of human virtuous activity,

> "There will be no danger of performing any evil action, since he practises temperance and despises money: all evil actions that men undertake are done either at the prompting of greed or under the spell of pleasure."[195]

Galen is optimistic that an improvement of moral conduct can be achieved through philosophical training and rational guidance of the irrational soul. In emphasising the corrective influence of reason and general philosophical doctrines,

190 Galen, *Soul's Dependence on the Body,* 172.
191 Autobiographical examples of such 'training of the soul' in Galen, *Affections and Errors of the Soul*, 118–120.
192 Galen, *Affections and Errors of the Soul*, 125.
193 Galen, *The Best Doctor is Also a Philosopher*, 32.
194 Jackson, *Doctors and Diseases in Roman Empire*, 57.
195 Galen, *The Best Doctor is Also a Philosopher*, 33–34.

Galen moves beyond a merely naturalist/functionalist or individualist account of health as developed by Boorse and Nordenfelt.

In his emphasis on the body-soul union as well as on rational training, he bridges contemporary philosophical approaches on the one hand (with their predominantly *exclusive* focus on the body or societal and cultural influences or the individual) and early Christian approaches on the other hand which seek to understand health in the context of an *inclusive* view of human life. Structurally not unlike Galen, early Christian writers sought to account for the patient as a person in the union of body and soul.

Yet unlike Galen, they did not understand this union *functionally* but *hierarchically*. They thought the soul needed improvement; unlike Galen they did not conceive of such improvement in rational and voluntary terms but thought that it could only be brought about God's gracious healing power. They were highly sceptical of any lasting and *real* improvement, not only of the human character or the soul, but also of the body on grounds of reason alone. Whilst the majority was interested in Galen's naturalist medicine and in philosophical training to varying degrees, they considered both medicine and philosophy as fragmentary approaches to human life and health, and on this basis as insufficient for achieving well-being or fullness of life. Christian theology focuses on this hope and its prolepsis signs in the present, not the temporal promises offered by medicine. A brief note on terminology (and beyond!): one can discuss whether early Christian writers were indeed theologians, or still (if not also) philosophers. As patristic scholar Wilhelm Geerlings remarks in *Theologians of Christian Antiquity,*[196]

> "Many [early Church] theologians figure in contemporary histories of philosophy. In late Antiquity philosophy and theology were not yet the neatly separated disciplines of the modern era – as if philosophy was based on pure reason alone, and theology restricted to penetrating God's revelation only."[197]

He continues,

> "It is pointless to ask whether an early Christian thinker should be best termed a philosopher or theologian. [...] Philosophy and theology penetrated each other; their interplay is *the* central aspect in the general process of Antiquity and Christendom."[198]

3.2 CONTEXTUALISING PATRISTIC WRITERS

The sheer number of healings said by the New Testament writers to be performed by Jesus, seems to suggest that the "phenomenon of healing [...] (was) a central factor in primitive Christianity".

The New Testament scholar, Howard C. Kee, explains further that the feature of healing does not appear simply as "an addendum to the tradition, introduced in

---

196 Geerlings (ed. 2002), *Theologen der christlichen Antike*. Here and in the following translations are my own.
197 Ibid., 7.
198 Ibid., 9.

order to make Jesus more appealing to the Hellenistic world"[199] but was "almost certainly a part of the historical core of that tradition, even though it is likely to have been embellished in the process of transmission."[200]

Before engaging with the early Christian fathers, I will look at the healing accounts that have a central position within the Gospel narratives. An emphasis will be on detailing the physical diseases mentioned with a view to their causes, the means through which healing was effected (e.g. miraculous healing or use of medical knowledge), as well as the explanatory theological horizon against which healing took place and wanted to be understood. I will engage with historians Vivian Nutton and Adolf von Harnack's rival examination of early Church attitudes to medicine. Whilst Nutton views the early Church as in competition with medical healers of the time, von Harnack concludes on the basis of his own analysis of historical sources that Christianity can be aptly described as a "medical religion" – that is, a religion open to, and intrinsically concerned with medical aspects of health and healing.

However, von Harnack also emphasises that Christianity's real concern with physical health can only be understood from within the eschatological promises of fullness of life – a view which indeed appears and reappears in the writings of the Church Fathers at the centre of this chapter. Both parts contextualise the early theologies of the Church. They introduce the ideas and types of arguments which Darrel W. Amundsen considered as propaedeutic to any "further discussion of the place of health, disease, healing and the art of medicine in early Christianity in general and in the theology of individual fathers in particular"[201] and which significantly bear upon the development of a theological understanding of the concept of health and the art of medicine which is the overall concern of this study. Embedding the writings of the Church Fathers in both scriptural and historical analysis will lead to a deeper understanding of the character of the ideas particular to Tatian, Tertullian, and Basil the Great.

3.2.1 The Gospel narratives: physical health and the coming kingdom

The phenomenon of healing is a central factor in early Christianity. At least forty-eight healing narratives can be found in the four gospels alone.[202] New Testament

---

199 Kee, *Medicine, Miracle, Magic*, 124.
200 Ibid.
201 Amundsen, *Body, Soul, Physician*, 6.
202 Sixteen healings can be found in the gospel according to Matthew, fourteen in Mark's and Luke's, and four in John's gospel. Below is a list of these key healing passages. References in brackets are, first, to the disease kind and, secondly, to particularities of healing. *Matthew:* 4:23-24 and 9:35 (general reference); 8:1 (man with a skin-disease, word); 8:5 (centurion's servant, word); 8:14 (Peter's mother-in-law, touch); 8:16 (devil possessed man, command); 9:1 (paralytic, forgiveness of sins and command); 9:18 (woman with a haemorrhage/official's daughter raised to life); 9:27 (two blind men, linking of faith and healing); 9:32 (demon possession); 12:9 (man with a withered hand; Sabbath healing); 12:22 (blind and dumb demoniac, forgiveness of sins); 15: 21 (Cannaanite woman, cleanliness); 15:29 (general reference);

scholar Howard C. Kee remarks in his 1986 *Medicine, Miracle and Magic in New Testament Times*,

> "Of the approximately 250 literary units into which the first three gospels are divided in a typical synopsis, one fifth either describe or allude to the healing and exorcist activities of Jesus and the disciples. Of the seven 'signs' reported in John to have been done by Jesus, four involve healing or restoration."[203]

Physical diseases range from temporary and rather harmless viral infections such as fever or influenza, to more severe and contagious skin-diseases, possibly of a leprous type, and to grave if not life-threatening afflictions such as blindness, epilepsy or paralysis. Demon possession counts as cause of disease. Yet demoniacs are always distinguished from those who suffer from those kinds of illnesses that are caused by, in medical terminology, natural infectious agents: in Matthew 8:16 the man possessed by devils is set apart from the rest of "all who were sick". Similarly, the healing account in Mark 1:32 sets apart those "who where sick" from "those who were possessed by devils."

Throughout the four gospels, the healing of physical affliction as well as demon possession is effected by Jesus (and later his followers, too) through touch or command, the latter either in the presence or absence of the afflicted. The choice of a particular healing mode appears random in so far as no apparent connections can be established: whilst it might be an obvious connection to link touch, for instance, with skin-diseases, it does not appear in the gospels; equally, more severe afflictions such as blindness are not connected with what might be seen as the more powerful of healing agents, the commanding word. Again, demon possession is an exception in as much as the only treatment mentioned is the driving out the evil spirit through command. The healing methods mentioned underline that the healings performed by Jesus were not based on the diagnostic or therapeutic knowledge of the time. Jesus is never portrayed as a doctor; he is no physician of his own intellectual power, or on the basis of his own medical knowledge and practical expertise. Neither theoretical reflections on the origin of diseases and disease classification, nor attention to treatment details are of particular interest to the evangelists. Instead they are accomplished through appeal to, and the subse-

---

17:14 (epileptic demoniac; link faith and healing); 21:14 (healing at the temple in Jerusalem). *Mark* (including parallel passages to Matthew/Luke): 1:23 (demoniac); 1:29 (Simon's mother-in-law); 1:32 (general sick and demoniacs); 1:40 (skin-disease); 2:1 (paralytic, forgiving of sins, faith); 3:1 (man with the withered hand, Sabbath); 5:1 (Gerasene demoniacs); 5:21 (man with haemorrhage, daughter of Jairus); 6:5 (general reference); 6:55 (several healings at Genesaret, touching the fringe of cloak); 7:24 (daughter of the Syro-Phoenician woman, cleanliness); 7:32 (deaf man); 8:22 (blind man at Bethsaida); 10:46 (blind man of Jericho, faith). *Luke* (again parallels to Mark and Matthew included): 4:31 (rebuking of a devil); 4:38 (Simon's mother-in-law); 4:40 (general healings); 5:12 (skin-disease); 5:17 (paralytic); 6:6 (withered hand, Sabbath); 7:1 (centurion's servant); 7:11 (son of the widow of Nain restored to life); 8 (woman with haemorrhage, Jairus' daughter); 9:37 (epileptic man); 13:10 (healing a crippled woman, Sabbath); 14:1 (dropsical man, Sabbath); 17:11 (skin-disease, faith); 22:49 (healing of the ear). *John:* 4:46 (the royal official's son); 5:2 (general healings); 9:1 (man born blind, Sabbath, sin and disease); 11:1 (Lazarus).
203 Kee, *Medicine, Miracle, Magic*, 1.

quent action of, God. Emphasis rests on the *end* of treatment, that is, the restoration of health set in the context of salvation.

As Kee says,

> "The healings and exorcisms are placed in a larger structure which sees what is happening as clues and foretastes of a new situation in which the purpose of God will finally be accomplished in the creation and his people will be vindicated and at peace."[204]

So, healing is not effected in reference to the laws of nature, but miraculously, through divine intervention; it is an event which occurs within human experience yet has not been "brought about by human power or by the operation of any natural agency and must therefore be ascribed to the special intervention of the Deity or of some supernatural being."[205]

According to Kee, miraculous healing *per definitionem* (yet not historically[206]) is sharply differentiated from medical healing, "a method of diagnosis of human ailments and prescription for them based on a combination of theory about and observation of the body, its functions and malfunctions"[207] and magic healing, a technique effective of itself[208] without need of divine or human intervention. Even though historically the boundaries of miraculous, medical, and magic healing tended to blur, the distinction is valid, for all three modes of healing presuppose and assume fundamentally different ideas of cosmic order and of human life in particular. Since Galen at least, medical healing builds upon the foundation of the regularity and order found in nature. Indeed, Kee refers to Galen's understanding of the medical art when he says

> "The goal of the physician is to discern the patterns of the natural functioning of the human body, by direct observation [...] by analogy [...] and by inference from philosophical principles of cosmic order which experience and reason have led him to adopt as normative."[209]

Magic healing through formulas or incantations, however common amongst healers and exorcists of the time, is not accounted for in the New Testament.[210] As Kee notes,

> "There is in the gospel narratives no trace of the elaborate multi-named invocations of the gods, the agglomerations of nonsense letters and syllables, the coercive manipulations of the unseen powers which characterise the magical papyri."[211]

Whilst neither explicitly condemning nor rejecting natural medicine, the gospel writers never appear greatly interested in specifically medical aspects of disease

---

204 Kee, *Medicine, Miracle, Magic*, 79.
205 Oxford English Dictionary, Vol. IX (1989), 835.
206 Kee, *Medicine, Miracle, Magic*, 3.
207 Ibid.
208 Ibid., 4.
209 Kee, *Medicine, Miracle, Magic*, 122.
210 Ibid., 79; cf. also 112–121. A more detailed account of the controversy over the question whether or not Jesus was a magician can not be given here – see for instance Smith, *Jesus the Magician* (1978); Hull, *Hellenistic Magic and the Synoptic Tradition* (1974); Gallagher, *Divine Man or Magician? Celsus and Origen on Jesus* (1981).
211 Cf. Kee, *Medicine, Miracle, Magic*, 126.

and treatment. Primarily, human diseases are of theological interest in that they are part of the burden weighing on 'fallen' human life. Healing and health anticipate the escheating, in which humans will be delivered both from bodily pain and spiritual disorder. This disinterest, even critical attitude[212] can be traced back to the Hebrew Bible where the Creator is depicted as sole restorer and ordered of individual, corporate human life[213] and where no human agency, least of all the agency of physicians, is described able to alleviate suffering or cure ills.[214]

Kee perceives a stark contrast between both kinds of healing when he says that they stand in two "fundamentally different frameworks of meaning"[215] with on the one hand the Christian view of the present reality as a foretaste of the new life in which God's creation and people will be vindicated and at peace, and on the other the medical view of natural reality as subject of rational, objectifiable observations and examinations, with purpose and order.

Yet notwithstanding this undeniable difference, for the New Testament writers physical healing in general, be it through medical or divine intervention, is placed within the context of the coming kingdom. Against this background, medical healing, too, heralds the new life and is a sign of the new aeon.[216] It is not a spectacle such as took place in the cults of Asclepius or Dionysius, but provides humans with the vision of eternal and inalienable wholeness and well-being which the gospels proclaimed. When Jesus returns to Galilee after the temptations in the desert, he announces the message of his ministry: repentance, forgiveness of sin, and the promise of the coming kingdom.[217] Here he starts his mission in words but also in deeds – first of all deeds of healing. Thus his message of repentance within the horizon of the coming kingdom is linked to the actions of healing:[218]

> "He went round the whole of Galilee teaching in their synagogues, proclaiming the good news of the kingdom and curing all kinds of disease and illness among the people. His fame spread throughout Syria, and those who were suffering from diseases and painful complaints of one kind or another, the possessed, epileptics, the paralysed were all brought to him, and he cured them."[219]

In the context of repentance and the announcement of the kingdom sense can be made of Sabbath healings.[220] According to Jewish *Halakhah*, the healing of minor injuries and afflictions on the Sabbath was an abrogation of the divine command to rest, from which exception could be made only in case of life-threatening illness. In the context of the coming kingdom, healing became a sign of God's saving grace in the eschatological future. Throughout the New Testament the em-

---

212 Mk 5:26; Lk 8:43; Lk 4:23.
213 Cf. book of Job, where advice of the comforters is dismissed as the deceit of liars and useless prescriptions of physicians; see also: II Chron 16:11-12; Jer 8:22-9:6; Jer 30:12-13 et al.
214 Kee, *Medicine, Miracle, Magic*, 17.
215 Ibid., 66.
216 Cf. John's Gospel 9:3 et. al. (use of the Greek term for sign 'semeia') and Acts 4:16, 8:6.
217 Mt 4:17 par.
218 Cf. Mt 9:35 par.
219 Mt 4:23 f. par.
220 Cf. Mt 12:9, Lk 6:6/13:10/14:1, Jn 9:1 et al.

phasis rests on the end of healing, namely the restoration of health through union with God. Theoretical or scientific reflection on the origin of diseases, any differentiation and classification of disease are of no interest. Whilst there are indications of a relation between disease and sin,[221] it is nowhere suggested that sin was the root of disease. Rather the opposite: a causality of disease and sin seems to be ruled out explicitly in the narrative of the cure of the man born blind.[222]

It is impossible to judge and assess the healing narratives from a mere medical or psychological standpoint. Nowhere in the New Testament can one find an outspoken condemnation of the art of medical healing; it is even recognised as a necessary body of knowledge.

This is what the use of Greek terms of medical healing such as '*therapeuo*' and '*iaomai*' suggests. Yet the frequent use of '*sozo*' with its etymological family '*soter/soteria*' points out that above all healing belongs to the theological message of humanity's salvation. Healing generally is described as visible sign of the alleviation of this burdensome evil, a sign of human reconciliation and redemption. Having its place within the order of salvation, medical healing is therefore one possible means of expression of grace.

3.2.2 Von Harnack: Christianity – a medical religion?

Given the early Church's concern with human well-being in its widest sense (namely that of salvation as shown above) and medicine's much more limited concern with bodily well-being, tensions and conflicts between the two might not be entirely unexpected. Historian of medicine Vivian Nutton remarks, "Christianity offered itself as direct competitor to secular healing."[223] It presented itself as the religion of not only spiritual well-being but also physical healing above all and *par excellence*. "In Christ, God incarnate, it had the saviour on earth, the great physician, whose help was available to all believers, and at no monetary costs."[224] The message of salvation linked up with physical health, and the performing of successful healings helped to secure Christianity's primacy among competing religions.[225]

A thesis similar to Nutton's had been put forward a hundred years earlier, at the end of the nineteenth century, yet from a perspective more sympathetic to the Christian cause. In his 1892 article "Medicinisches aus Ältester Kirchengeschich-

---

221 Mk 2:5 par.; Jn 5:14.
222 Jn 9:1 f. This interpretation is in contrast to the account of the Hebrew Bible, where sickness and death are often interpreted as God's punishment for human disobedience to his will. Cf. Num. 12:9, Deut. 28:15, 1 Kings 14:1–18, Ps 38:3–9 et.al. See also: Allan, *Physician in Ancient Israel*, 377–378.
223 Nutton, "Murders and Miracles", 48–49.
224 Ibid.
225 Ibid.

te"[226] the German theologian Adolf von Harnack looked at the relationship of ancient medicine and early Christianity, and the ways in which the example of Jesus
Christ and his apostles influenced medical practice of the first centuries. Von
Harnack's position differs from Nutton's in so far as he denies the (in some disciplines still prevailing) assumption of an inherent suspicion of, and competition or
hostility between, medicine and Christianity. He confirms an understanding of
Christianity as concerned with physical healing but with in view the positive implications for the development of Western medicine as we know it today.

In concluding, von Harnack formulates his perhaps rather unexpected thesis
of Christianity as a "medical religion."[227] This for him includes the almost universal positive recognition of natural medicine as Galen practised it. In characterising
the Christian religion as "medical", von Harnack goes beyond the view that described Christianity as a religion concerned primarily with health and healing in a
spiritual sense.[228] In coining the term "medical religion" he disputed the view of
an antithetical or disinterested relationship of Christianity and secular medicine.

Von Harnack sets out to defend Christianity at a time of an increasing interpretative importance of the natural sciences. He claims an *intrinsic* link between
natural medicine and Christianity, and establishes this link in offering an account
of Christian physicians of the first centuries, ranging from Luke the evangelist to
the two brothers and patron saints of medicine, Cosmas and Damian, and compris-
ing more than a dozen commonly unknown Christian physicians of the Greco-
Roman world.[229] He also lists and details recognised dietetic and therapeutic
measures mentioned in the New Testament[230] and by the early Christian writers.[231] Indeed, as von Harnack shows, the writings of the early Church Fathers
from both East and West contain an astonishing number of texts on physiology,
psychology, epidemiology and nosology[232] in the light of which the often-reported
belief in demons and exorcism can be submitted to critical review.[233]

When directing the reader's attention to the gospels' account of Jesus' healings in the last chapter of his article, von Harnack underlines that these took place
within a world craving for health and healing. Both the philosophy and medicine
of the Roman Empire did not procure sufficient response to suffering to the effect
that people began to look for consolation and salvation in religious healing cult.
The increased popularity of the cult of Asclepius, the *deus clinicus,* vouches for
this increased interest in religion in the context of diseases. For von Harnack, this

---

226 "Medical ideas in the history of the early Church" (Here and in the following translations are
my own).
227 Harnack, Medicinisches aus Ältester Kirchengeschichte, 132 ("medizinische Religion").
228 As will be shown below such a view is not entirely beside the point where early Church theologians underlined the hierarchical order of body and soul, distinguished between bodily and
spiritual health, and valued the latter higher in so far as it leads to union with God and eternal
salvation.
229 Harnack, Medicinisches aus Ältester Kirchengeschichte, 37–50.
230 1. Tim 5:23.
231 Harnack, Medicinisches aus Ältester Kirchengeschichte, 51–67.
232 Ibid., 67–104.
233 Ibid., 105–124.

general longing for well-being and the view of a religion as a power able to bring about health was most certainly the crucial reason for Christianity's wide acceptance and final victory within a pagan environment: it established Christianity as a medical religion.[234]

In his article, von Harnack explores *historically* the relationship between Christianity and a medicine that is based on the knowledge of natural processes and the principles of logical analysis, experience, hypothesis and testing through experiments. Yet any compilation of historical material, he concedes, is only moved beyond the accidental if viewed in the context of the New Testament's gospel of Jesus Christ who promised and brought healing for humanity,[235] and through the grace of the spirit who locates the past in the present of our experience. In other words, the relationship between medicine and Christianity needs to be viewed *theologically* in light of the New Testament's message of salvation. The promise of salvation includes the restoration of human life in its unity of body and soul. And it is the distinct knowledge of human life as fallen, finite, at the same time redeemed and under the promise of eternal life that teaches humans about medicine's possibilities and limitations.

3.3 NATURAL MEDICINE AND DEMONIC POWERS: TATIAN

Of Tatian's writings only the *Oratio ad Graecos* and a synopsis of the four gospels, *Diatessaron*, have survived, which considerably restricts any inquiry as to his thinking. I focus here on Tatian's critique of pharmacology as presented in the *Oratio*. Pharmacology, one of the three branches of second century medicine (the others being dietetics and surgery), is rejected as an art that uses material substances to cure diseases. For Tatian, material substances are manifestations of demonic powers dwelling in nature (and so are physical diseases). His critique is rooted in his anthropology and understanding of creation, which he sets out to explain in the *Oratio* (chapters 12 to 15).

Tatian's account of a theological anthropology is essentially soteriological and pneumatological. It omits Christology almost entirely.[236] Tatian focuses on the relation of *matter* and *spirit(s)* in humans – a relation, which is foundational for his critique of pharmacology or perhaps medicine more generally (chapters 16 to 18).

I look first at Tatian's understanding of the goodness of matter in union with the spirit and above all the particularities of the divine (or holy) spirit. Its separation from the body after the Fall allows for the entry of demons into the body, which cause all kinds of diseases. I turn to pharmacology and involvement of demons both in diseases and cures. The connection of demons to diseases as well as

---

234 Harnack, "Medicinisches aus Ältester Kirchengeschichte", 132.
235 Ibid., 125.
236 Hauschild, *Gottes Geist und Mensch*, 206. For the problem of reception of Tatian cf. Amundsen, *Medicine, Society, Faith*, 159.

drugs calls for a Christian rejection of pharmacology, Tatian concludes. It remains subject to debate whether Tatian's views can be taken as rejecting medicine as a whole (that is, inclusive of surgery and dietetics) or only pharmacology as one of its parts. Clearly, Tatian's vehement critique of pharmacological cures does not leave room for practical recommendations other than *avoid drugs* – and perhaps medicine altogether. The final section assesses whether Tatian's position is the extreme view of an outsider or whether it found wider support within the tradition of early Christianity.

3.3.1 Hierarchical union of matter, soul, and the divine spirit

"The whole construction and creation of the world has derived from matter, and ... matter has itself been produced by God in such a way that we are to think of it partly as raw and form-less before its separation, partly as organized and orderly after its division."[237]

The world *is* matter, and God *makes* matter. Hence, matter cannot be alien or op-posed to God's being, which is the absolute good, Tatian concludes. However, he continues, "This being so, there are differences among material things, so that one is better, another good in itself but inferior to something superior."[238] With regard to the human body, there are also gradations of goodness yet overall there is "harmonious agreement." In Tatian's own words,

"There are certain grades of honour in it. One part is an eye, another an ear, another a particu-lar kind of hair arrangement, or ordering of the intestines, or conjunction of bone and marrow and sinew; *and although one part differs from another, in the overall plan there is harmoni-ous agreement.*"[239]

In unity with matter there exists in the world a spirit: a "spirit in luminaries, spirit in angels, spirit in plants and waters, spirit in men, and spirit in animals."[240] This spirit is one and the same but also possesses "differences within itself."[241] The material spirit (*pneuma hylikon*) or "soul"[242] exists in all beings; it penetrates the material world thus forming a union of spirit and matter. The human body and soul are such a union. The soul "can never appear by itself apart from the body, nor is the flesh resurrected apart from the soul."[243] This "material spirit" is not in itself immortal but mortal.[244]

Yet humans, Tatian writes, were not always bodily matter and material spirit only. Originally, they possessed a third component, the *divine spirit*. This divine

237 Tatian, *Oratio ad Graecos*, 12; 4; 5.
238 Ibid., 12.
239 Ibid. (my italics).
240 Ibid.
241 Ibid.
242 Ibid.
243 Tatian, *Oratio ad Graecos*, 15. The belief in a bodily resurrection militates against a classifi-cation of matter as evil. Cf. chapter four, Augustine on the importance of Christ's resurrection for the recognition and affirmation of the goodness of bodily existence.
244 Tatian, *Oratio ad Graecos*, 13.

spirit was "greater than the soul."[245] It was "the image"[246] or "knowledge"[247] of God. In being the image it was different from both the Creator himself and from his divine logos. Tatian calls the divine spirit also the "holy spirit" (*to pneuma to agion*)[248] without, however, developing the dogmatic of a distinctively Christian pneumatology or a doctrine of the Trinity which was not formulated until 200 years later.[249] The divine spirit is on one level with the transcendent divine nature of God without being a distinct person in the sense formulated by the council of Nicaea.[250]

For Tatian's anthropology, as well as the present context, it is necessary to understand that the divine spirit used to be the soul's companion, "but gave it up when the soul was unwilling to follow it"[251] in the events reported in the first chapters of the book of Genesis. Fallen humanity is severed from the Holy Spirit, which is the reason for its being subject to sin and death. Humans can acquire immortality only if they gain back the union of the material and the divine spirit: for only then the material spirit "mounts to the realms above where the spirit leads it; for the spirit's home is above, but the soul's birth is below."[252]

The union may be regained in faith and through repentance, Tatian says.[253] Even after the Fall God is willing to dwell through the divine spirit, his "representative"[254] as Peter Brown put it.

However, where the union of matter and the divine spirit remains lost, humans are mere *torsoi*. Being inhabited by the divine spirit is what makes humans *human* beings and distinct from animals. In itself, the human soul is nothing; it exists – in Brown's words – "to be married to the spirit."[255] In this, Tatian's anthropology stresses "the 'vertical' dimension of the human person. The joining of the existing, insufficient human being to the Holy Spirit formed the centre of gravity of his thought."[256] Souls that do not cleave to the divine spirit "must fall into an equally intimate and all-engulfing state of possession by the spirits of evil."[257]

---

245 Tatian, *Oratio ad Graecos*, 12.
246 Ibid.
247 Ibid., 13.
248 Ibid., 15.
249 Cramer, *Geist Gottes in frühsyrischer Theologie*, 52.
250 Ibid., 57.
251 Tatian, *Oratio ad Graecos*, 13.
252 Ibid.
253 Ibid., 15.
254 Brown, *Body and Society*, 91
255 Ibid.
256 Ibid., 90.
257 Ibid., 91.

3.3.2 Demonic involvement in diseases and medicinal drugs

Diseases are demons' visitations on human bodies.[258] The demons bring about changes in bodily matter. Bodily matter, which is not bad in itself, becomes evil under the influence of evil spirits, and then needs to be rejected.[259] They are signs of a body's possession by evil spirits where the body has become vulnerable to their attack due to its post-fallen dissociation from the divine spirit.

Demons do not possess "a particle of flesh"[260] but are of spiritual constitution like fire or air.[261] They are malign beings that rage against humans. At times, Tatian views them as fallen angels which became pagan gods.[262]

Medicinal drugs used for the treatment of diseases are material, too; they are either produced by doctors who use material knowledge (thus act on behalf of the demons) or prescribed by pagan gods who are themselves former demons. Tatian rejects all medical drugs not because they are material but because they are demonic in origin.

> "The varieties of roots and applications of sinews and bones are not efficacious in themselves; they are the elemental matter of the demons' wickedness, which produce effects in the areas where they have determined that each of these should be individually potent."[263]

Darrel W. Amundsen concludes that demons for Tatian are subtle deceivers.

> "Especially rankling for Tatian would be the self-assurance that the naturalist (like Galen) and those who administer or take medicinal drugs display by thinking that the drugs are within their control and subordinate to their lofty intellects."[264]

According to Tatian, demons use diseases (and the cures thereof) for the enslavement of humans.[265] They allow certain products of nature (hence, material products) to be efficient so that humans become dependent upon them and grow distracted from God on whom alone they depend. "Whenever they see that men have accepted service by using these means they seduce them and make them their slaves."[266] As a consequence, to rely on "herbs and roots"[267] offered by doctors or temple priests in the service of demons is to turn away from God and towards evil spirits or demons. Here, humans forsake the possibility of re-uniting their bodies and material spirits with the divine spirit. Being inhabited by the divine spirit is what makes humans *human* beings and distinct from animals. As such, natural remedies lower human beings to the level of animals:

> "Why is the man who puts his faith in the material system unwilling to trust in God? For what reason do you not resort to the lord of superior power, but choose rather to heal yourself like a

258 Tatian, *Oratio ad Graecos*, 17/18.
259 Ibid., 16.
260 Ibid., 15.
261 Ibid.
262 Ibid., 16.
263 Ibid., 17.
264 Amundsen, *Medicine, Society, Faith*, 168.
265 Tatian, *Oratio ad Graecos*, 17.
266 Ibid.
267 Ibid.

dog with grass, or a deer with a snake, a hog with river crabs, or a lion with monkeys? Why, pray, do you make gods out of this world's things?"[268]

3.3.3 Concluding remarks

According to Tatian, matter is not inherently evil. Yet where dissociated from the spirit, it is susceptible and subject to perversion. It may become an instrument of evil, as is the case both in diseases and medical (pharmacological) treatment. Only God's word can heal for it forces the demons to disappear. In re-uniting the body with the divine spirit, it frees humans to be *truly human*.

> "Now there are diseases and disorders of the matter within us, but the demons take credit for these whenever they occur, and follow sickness wherever it strikes. Sometimes too they shake the body's system with a fit of their own madness, and then smitten by a word of God's power they go away in fear and the sick man is healed."[269]

Tatian suggests a relation between demons and disease, or the supernatural and the natural, not between sin and disease, which is an important difference with regard to his position as a Christian writer. In this view, he follows the New Testament writers' rejection of the former and acceptance of the latter.[270]

He condemns both medical pharmacology (which would not be efficient, if the demons did want it to be thus) and the temple cures of the cult of Asclepius (which as pagan cult cures are demonic in origin). Tatian's hostility to pharmacology as a branch of medicine "was not the result of his heretical inclinations but of his quite orthodox, though extreme, demonology"[271] and was then more a question of emphasis, and not of doctrinal innovation or eccentricity. In his critique of pharmacology, he does not explicitly refer to Galen but to one of the branches of the naturalist kind of medicine which Galen epitomised.

Despite the vehemence of his criticism, historians of medicine Owsei Temin[272] and Darrel W. Amundsen agree that Tatian's *Oratio* can not be read as an outright condemnation of medicine *per se*.[273] Amundsen even goes so far as to place Tatian's criticism within the context of a *medical* critique of pharmacology that emanated amongst certain groups of physicians of the time.

> "Even though Galen and others insisted on the unity of the three parts of medicine (pharmacology, dietetics, and surgery), not all physicians and laymen agreed. There was no unanimity

---

268 Tatian, *Oratio ad Graecos*, 18.
269 Ibid.
270 An early link between sickness, death and demons might be seen in *The Book of Tobit* (2nd century BC). In the first century AD, Josephus and Philo mention the belief in the link between demons and sickness at least for the Qumran sect, the Essenes. Partly replacing the connection of sickness and sin, suffering and disabilities are regarded as the word of Satan and his cohorts (cf. Kee, *Medicine, Miracle, Magic*, 21–26).
271 Amundsen, "Medicine and Faith in Early Christianity", 346/350. Cf. Elze, *Tatian*, 100–103.
272 Temkin, *Hippocrates in a World of Pagan and Christians*, 122.
273 Amundsen, *Medicine, Society and Faith*, 159.

of opinion among the various medical sects regarding the proper use of drugs. Some physicians rejected their use altogether."[274]

Amundsen notes that Tatian agreed with the majority of the Church Fathers in not putting one's faith in medicine. However, he went further in considering one part of medicine as especially dangerous. In pharmacology the involvement of demons is often too subtle to be recognised, particularly when cloaked in the language of philosophical naturalism or (Galenic) rationalism.[275] For Tatian pharmacology is dangerous not for the reasons a physician would give but *spiritually*. This is, of course, where his critique differs from criticism that arose within the medical community of his times.

Referring to the early Church more generally, Amundsen says that three positive and negative attitudes towards medicine can be distinguished. The three positive include (1) the view of creation of the world as good and of all material substance; (2) the view of created nature as a reservoir of God's providential care for humans; and (3) the view of medicine based on human knowledge of nature as an art beneficial for humanity. The negative principles point out (1) the limitations on the occasions on which Christians should use the services of medicine; (2) the sources of healing other than God – e.g. demons; and (3) possible misuse of the art of medicine in the hands of (fallen) humans.[276] And it is in the latter sense that the writings (and warnings!) of Tatian need to be understood.

Tatian's interest is in the *vertical* dimension of human life, the relationship of the body to the human soul to the divine (or holy) spirit, and that its leads to true human-ness. The union of body-soul-divine spirit is a hierarchical union with the divine spirit being the highest and most important for human well-being. Tatian sees his task as one of warning against demonic deception.

Tatian's concern is with enabling true human flourishing in relationship with the Creator. For Tatian, human-ness can be realised only where the supernatural in humans (that is, the divine soul) is subordinated to God and where it rules the natural from a position of moral superiority. The natural un-ruled is open to misuse by evil supernatural powers (that is, demons) that seek to infringe upon matter. Demons cause diseases, and are behind medicinal drugs, which they use as a way of enslaving humans, of making them dependent upon their evil mastery. Thus they prevent human beings from living in real human-ness; they reduce them to an animal state. Above all, according to Tatian, humans should be concerned with what it means to be living a *human* life, not a *healthy* life. And since this question can only be answered in referring to God and his word, who alone is the first and superior master of the body-soul union, hence of health, *human* life also means well-being within its earthly limitations.

Tertullian, Tatian's contemporary from the Latin-speaking West of the Roman Empire, shared his concern with *true* human-ness and well-being as of first and foremost importance. In Tertullian's thought, this concern is present above all

---

274 Amundsen, *Medicine, Society and Faith*, 163.
275 Ibid., 170
276 Amundsen, *Body, Soul, Physician*, 6–8.

in his distinction of spiritual and physical health, and in his treatment of the sacrament of baptism. However, Tertullian recognised deficiencies in nature as one possible cause of human diseases, and medical knowledge as one possible means of restoring physical health. In Tertullian, the doors for medicine are if not open then at least ajar.

3.4 HIERARCHY OF PHYSICAL AND SPIRITUAL HEALTH: TERTULLIAN

Tertullian pioneered the Latinisation of Christian discourse. He was the first significant Christian author to write entirely in Latin, even though fluently mastering Greek. His profound knowledge of philosophy as well as his preoccupation with the relationship of Christian faith and Greek philosophy are his distinguishing features within Patristic theology. He is well known for the alleged claim that philosophy and theology had nothing in common. What has Athens to do with Jerusalem? Tertullian is reported to have once exclaimed. What has the Academy in common with the church? Due to this famous question being attributed to him, Tertullian is commonly understood to have drawn a sharp line between Christian truth and philosophical pronouncements.[277]

> "Almost every word he wrote gave the lie to the answer he implies. [...] He explicitly rejected a Stoic, Platonic or dialectical Christianity. But in a wider sense, he had himself reconciled Christianity and classical culture. He used the benefits of a traditional education and the fruits of his pagan erudition to defend and to propagate what he considered to be the truth."[278]

Tertullian's attitude towards medicine and its underlying philosophical tenets gives testimony to an approach that is of a more conjoining than divisive nature. He saw human reason as God's gift. He cautiously recommended medicine, the study of nature and of rational theorems on human bodily functioning.[279]

However, considering the little room Tertullian allows for the discussion of physical disease and medical healing in his work, it seems appropriate to say that physical health does not seem to be of predominant importance for overall well-being.

Given his interest in, and knowledge of, philosophical works, it seems plausible to assume that he had heard of Galen's epistemology and some medical tenets of his time. Yet he does not engage with them, nor does he refer to medical epistemology as tools for finding out about disease symptoms and therapeutic measures. Tertullian thought that physical diseases could stem from natural entities affecting the body. Yet more importantly, they may be caused by demonic interferences in the body or may have a spiritual cause such as heretical belief.

Disease causality is marked by the interplay of supernatural forces and nature. Where diseases have their origin in an external infliction on bodily nature, the patient requires knowledge of natural processes; where demons are behind phys-

---

277 See for instance Harakas, *Health in the Orthodox Tradition*, 70.
278 Barnes, "Tertullian", 210.
279 Tertullian, *Chaplet*, chapters 3–4.

ical ailment they need to be exorcised through the power of God's word; where disease is caused by wrong belief, humans need to turn to God as present in the sacraments of his Church.

Tertullian's treatment of the sacrament of baptism shows (a) his analogous use of physical disease and medicine and (b) his view of spiritual health as of greater value. Spiritual health alone leads to eternal flourishing and true human fulfilment, which Tertullian understood to be human life's ultimate end. In recognising to a limited degree natural disease causes and naturalist medicine, Tertullian qualifies medicine as a beneficial art. However, it is never sufficient for human well-being. Tertullian's emphasis is always on the spiritual dimension of human life.

3.4.1 On disease causes: natural, demonic, and spiritual

In the *Antidote to the Scorpion's Bite*, Tertullian introduces the distinction between physical and spiritual disease in relation to disease causes, as well as the analogous usage of disease language and medical healing in the dealing with heretical belief and divine cures.

On one level, the *Antidote* deals with the physical effects of the toxic sting of scorpions and the required medical treatment. Tertullian describes in detail the scorpion and its (often) life-threatening bite:

> "That succession of knots in the scorpion, which in the inside is a thin poisoned veinlet, rising up with a bow-like bound, draws tight a barbed sting at the end, after the manner of an engine for shooting missiles."[280]

Yet of course, his aim is nowhere to advance or contribute to existing medical work on scorpion's bites, nor does he engage further with medical disease knowledge or therapies.

Instead, he is concerned above all with spiritual wounds and inflictions caused by the poisoning belief of the Gnostic sect. The discussion of external, physical wounds caused by the real entity of the scorpion is used analogously for the more important internal, spiritual wounds and the religious cures required. Scorpions are metaphors for Gnostic believers; their venom is heretical belief; the poison's effect on the body is analogous to the wounds to the human soul, for which the only remedy is God, the supreme Physician. God alone is endowed with power over the human soul and will therefore provide help against the spiritual poison of the Gnostic heresy. He heals with his word which is like a medical drink. In Tertullian's words,

> "You who read will at the same time drink. Nor is the draught bitter. If the utterances of the Lord are sweeter than honey and the honey-combs, the juices are from that source. If the promise of God flows with milk and honey, the ingredients which go to make that draught have the smack of this."[281]

---

280 Tertullian, *Antidote*, 1.
281 Ibid.

Tertullian treated the possibility of demon-caused illnesses in his *Apology*. In reference to Gen 6:1–4 and in accordance with many of his contemporaries, he saw demons as the offspring of corrupted angels.

> "Some of the angels, of their own accord, were perverted and then constituted the source of the even more corrupt race of devils, a race damned by God together with the originators of the race and him whom we have mentioned as their leader, the account is found in Sacred Scripture."[282]

The aim of the fallen creatures is the corruption of humanity, which may take the form of diseases as well as sudden changes of mood, eruptions of an unbalanced, restless spirit or turning away from contemplation of God. Demons effect a corruption that influences both body and soul.[283] In the same sense,

> "It is with the same mysterious power of infection that the breath of demons and [fallen] angels induces the corruption of the mind by foul passions, by dread derangements of the mind, or by savage lusts accompanied by manifold perversities."[284]

Both kinds of injuries, spiritual and physical, may be willed by God as a trial of faith. If the trial is overcome, human faith may be strengthened for strength can be perfected in weakness.[285] God might choose to use the scorpion or demons to inflict painful and seemingly unjust injuries for "he has chosen to contend with a disease and to do good by imitating the malady [...] to aid the flesh by injuring it, to preserve the soul by snatching it away."[286]

Natural or supernatural entities, injustice and pain are the instruments with which this trial is brought about. However, God himself is not unjust: out of justice, he uses the evil instrument of injustice to lead humans to his justice. Injustice comes to pass by the devil's agency, yet this is fundamentally different from saying that it originates in the devil's will in opposition to God's will and intentions.[287] God is good and he is the only ruler of the world, of nature and demons alike. Acting on behalf of God in a trial of faith, demons need to be overcome through faith. In other words, not only spiritual but also physical afflictions may be cured through the power of faith.

3.4.2 Modes of healing: natural, supernatural, and sacramental

Three modes of healing (sacramental, miraculous and medical) correspond to the three causes of disease (spiritual, demonic and natural). Illness caused by demons is healed through God's divine power evoked for instance in exorcisms. Though supporting miraculous and medical healing which effect temporal cures, Tertul-

---

282 Tertullian, *Apology*, 22/3.
283 Ibid., 22/4–5.
284 Ibid., 22/6–7.
285 Tertullian, *Flight*, all of chapter 2.
286 Tertullian, *Antidote*, 5.
287 Tertullian, *Flight*, all of chapter 2.

lian's treatment of the sacrament of baptism shows that ultimately spiritual health and healing are to be ranked higher.

The previous section allowed for three distinctions. Diseases can be caused by (1) natural entities, (2) demons, or (3) heretical belief. Three kinds of healing correspond to the three causes of illness: physical illness as deficiency of nature requires medicine's knowledge based upon the observation of nature; physical illness caused by demons requires exorcism; and spiritual illness (possibly intermingled with physical affliction) requires sacramental healing.

(1) Tertullian's acceptance of medicine is rooted in the conviction that God has revealed himself as the one who is endowed with *all* healing power. Medical healing is part of God's plan for humankind's salvation. Physicians are God's instruments in an operation that aims at humankind's wholeness. To employ medicine is a way of praising the author of this tool of healing. In this context Tertullian sharply disapproves of certain of his fellows, who would rather die than rely on medical knowledge. Such rejection is a rejection of God's intentions for humankind.[288] The therapeutic measures of medicine might "have an apparent cruelty, by reason of the lancet, and of the burning iron, and of the great heat of the mustard"[289] yet one should not oppose to them because they partake in God's restoration of human body *and* soul.

(2) In relating to that which is *above* nature, physical disease caused by demons cannot be overcome through medical treatment based on the observation *of* nature. The power of exorcism, which rests on the divine power that surpasses reason, imagination and understanding, has been handed by the Father to the Son and then to the disciples so that, in Tertullian's words,

> "At a touch, a breath from us, rebuked by the thought and description of that fire, at our command, they quit the bodies of men – but against their will and grieving and blushing because you are present."[290]

In *The Antidote*, Tertullian offers another example of how supernatural healing can be performed: as confession of faith, one makes the sign of the cross over the wounded part, then adjures the part in the name of Jesus and finally covers the poisoned part with "the gore of the beast when it has been crushed to death."[291]

The restoration of the body or its parts is not explained with reference to processes of nature. It is a marvellous event which well occurs within human experience yet has not been "brought about by human power or by the operation of any natural agency and must therefore be ascribed to the special intervention of the Deity or of some supernatural being"[292] so that it may be termed *miracle* healing.

(3) Whilst recognising the reality of bodily harm and inflictions independently of supernatural interferences, and accepting medicine as a mode of cure, too, in his work on *Baptism* Tertullian makes it clear that before anything else humans

---

288 Tertullian, *Antidote*, 5.
289 Ibid.
290 Tertullian, *Apology*, 23/16.
291 Tertullian, *Antidote*, 1.
292 *Oxford English Dictionary*, Vol. IX, 835.

should be concerned with their spiritual wounds, and should seek healing through God's sacraments in the first place: these are the highest forms of healing.

Tertullian begins by explaining first the more general meaning of water and its effective healing power in the light of both the Old and New Testament before going on to the ritual of baptism and the ultimate significance of baptismal healing in the light of Jesus Christ's passion and resurrection.

Throughout Antiquity, water was considered to interfere with human well-being. It was well known as the source of certain diseases, amongst which malaria was probably the most frequent. The author of the treatise *Airs, Waters, Places* belonging to the Hippocratic Corpus distinguishes different kinds of water, relates them to the seasonal changes of climate and gives an account of the resulting diseases.[293] Yet characteristic for the Hippocratic Corpus (and this in contrast to widely held opinions) is the refusal to accept supernatural interference with water as reason for physical disease.

Against the natural-medical tradition sketched here, Tertullian conceived of interplay of nature and the supernatural world: spirits may inhabit waters and cause its distinctively different qualities. He refers this claim to the beginning of the world when the general goodness of water was affirmed, for the spirit of God was said to reside upon the waters.[294] In the world after the Fall, unclean spirits can settle upon waters, "pretending to reproduce that primordial resting of the divine Spirit upon them."[295] This can have a negative effect for everyone in geographical proximity "as witness shady springs and all sorts of unfrequented streams, pools in bathing-places, and channels or storage-tanks in houses and those wells called snatching-wells – obviously they snatch by the violent action of a malignant spirit."[296] Clean spirits can settle upon waters and cause beneficial changes in nature: John 5:4 talks about the healing effects of the pool of Bethsaida, which was stirred once a year through angelic powers. The first man who stepped into the pool after the stirring of the water recovered from whatever temporal infirmity it was that oppressed him. "Those who complained of ill-health used to watch out for him, for anyone who got down there before the others, after washing had no further reason to complain."[297] These examples prove the presence of spirits, both good and bad ones, in normal water as in the water of baptism. The *temporal* healing of the *body* in the waters of Bethsaida is prophetic and illustrative of the *eternal* healing of the *spirit* in the waters of baptism "by the general rule that carnal things always come first as examples of things spiritual."[298]

> "As the grace of God makes general progress, both the waters and the angel have obtained more power. They used to remedy bodily defects, but now heal the spirit: they used to administer temporal health, but now restore the health which is eternal: they used to set free one

---

293 Hippocratic Writings, *Airs, Waters, Places*, pp. 152–155.
294 Gen. 1: 2.
295 Tertullian, *Baptism*, 5.
296 Ibid.
297 Ibid.
298 Ibid.

man, once a year, but now every day save nations, destroying death by the washing away of sins."[299]

Both the temporal healing of Bethsaida and the spiritual healing of baptism are caused by God's gracious power. However, in Bethsaida, humans were cured from bodily defects only. They merely gained temporal health. In baptism, post-fallen guilt is washed away entirely to the effect that the penalty of spiritual death is removed.

Evidently as the guilt is removed the penalty also is taken away. In this way man is being restored to God, to the likeness of him who had aforetime been in God's image – the image had its actuality in the man God formed, the likeness becomes actual in eternity – for there is given back to him the spirit of God which of old he had received of God's breathing, but afterwards had lost through sin.[300]

3.4.3 Concluding remarks

In the *Antidote to the Scorpion's Bite*, Tertullian introduced the distinction of physical and spiritual disease, as well as the analogous usage of disease language and medical therapies in the dealing with heretical belief and divine cures. He expounded physical and spiritual diseases as hierarchically ordered according to the gravity of risk involved for overall human well-being. Both kinds of diseases may entail death, yet spiritual death is to be ranked above physical death for it is the dissolution of one's relationship with God. Spiritual diseases are caused by wrong belief. Physical wounds may be caused by natural living entities such as the scorpion (and then have their place in nature alone) yet also by supernatural entities such as demons (and then result from the interplay of nature and the supernatural sphere).

However, the boundaries here are fuzzy since demons might act as scorpions in disguise. Like Tatian, Tertullian did not perceive clear boundaries between the natural and the supernatural as is underlined by his understanding of both natural and supernatural entities as God's tools: they may be willed and used by God to save the human soul. He "has chosen to contend with a disease and to do good by imitating the malady [...] (he) aids the flesh by injuring it, to preserve the soul by snatching it away."[301]

Notwithstanding Tertullian's emphasis on the interplay of nature and the supernatural, his recognition of the natural as good, and of diseases as also caused by natural entities allowed him to accept medical healing as good. Even more so, since he considered the art of medicine as belonging to, and expressing, God's salvific plan for humanity. To employ medicine is a way of praising the author of this tool of healing. In comparison with Tatian's critique of pharmacology, one can say that Tertullian left the doors to medicine a little further ajar.

---

299 Tertullian, *Baptism*, 5.
300 Ibid.
301 Tertullian, *Antidote*, 5.

At the same time, the continuous interplay of nature and the supernatural limits the practical relevance of medical therapies: where a physical disease has its cause in a demonic interference, medical cures fail to be effective in their dealings with visible bodily symptoms.

Natural knowledge might allow for the alleviation of pain and symptoms, yet it cannot eradicate the disease at its roots where these stem from the supernatural sphere, which medicine cannot access and understand. In relating to that which is *above* nature, physical disease caused by demons cannot be overcome through medical treatment based on the observation of that which is *within* and *of* nature.

Whilst recognising the reality of bodily harm and inflictions independently of supernatural interferences, and accepting medicine as one possible mode of cure, in *On Baptism* Tertullian underlined that above all humans should be concerned with their spiritual wounds. They should seek freedom from demons, and *spiritual* healing through God's sacraments. Medical healing is indeed *a good* yet for the reasons given in the context of the sacrament of baptism, Tertullian speaks about it as *less of a good* than spiritual healing. Medical healing based on natural knowledge is subordinated to God's healing power. It is a secondary mode of healing.

The use of medicine as store of analogies for the description and explanation of spiritual events fits into this assessment, too. In saying that temporal health might serves as means of illustrating spiritual health, and that medicine provides analogies for the spirit's health, Tertullian demonstrated again medicine's subordination to theology. Medicine is a means to an end in so far as it helps to explain the higher mode of healing, which is spiritual. Tertullian saw the body as a stage where nature and the supernatural meet and interact.

This view, in combination with his hierarchical understanding of the body's union with the soul, allowed him to recognise medicine and to limit it at the same time by pointing out the greater importance of spiritual health, which is relationship with God, the Creator. Tertullian's tentative approach to medicine does not allow for in-depth reflection on medical morality. Like Tatian's, his concern is with human well-being more generally. Here, spiritual health is more important than the freedom of physical symptoms or socio-personal aspects of human existence.

The idea of interplay between nature and evil spirits was rejected by fourth century Greek Father Basil the Great. This allowed him to support medical knowledge and practice, which he also saw as an art given to humanity by God so that it may foster and restore health. Basil's recognition of medicine invited him to reflect on medical practice in the context of the good life. The next section looks at Basil's account of disease, health, and medical healing and the practical implications of his reflection on medical practice from the perspective of the good life as exemplified in the active life of Jesus Christ.

3.5 MEDICAL PRACTICE AND CHARITY: BASIL THE GREAT

Amongst patrologists, Basil the Great (330–379), bishop of Caesarea, Gregory of Nazianzus, his friend, and Gregory of Nyssa, his brother, are known as the Cappadocian Fathers. They continued the work of the Alexandrian Father Athanasius (295–373) and aimed to overthrow the Arian doctrines in Asia Minor, hence, to defend the faith of Nicaea and to preserve the unity of the Church.[302] Though the three are united by their common theological and ecclesiastical interests as well as

> "By the bonds of a close and life-long friendship, each one of them represents a different type of personality. Thus, Basil is known as the man of action, Gregory of Nazianzus as the master of oratory and Gregory of Nyssa as the thinker."[303]

Only Basil is attributed the cognomen *great*, the great American patrologist Johannes Quasten remarks:

> "His outstanding qualifications as an ecclesiastical statesman and organiser, as a great exponent of Christian doctrine and as a second Athanasius in the defence of orthodoxy, as the Father of oriental monasticism and reformer of the liturgy, warrant the conferring of such a title."[304]

To add to Quasten's list, Basil, "the man of action" studied medicine himself, and is considered in the history of medicine as the founder of the first hospital of the Western world.[305] He showed great appreciation of those who followed the medical profession, of which he himself had gained knowledge while studying in Athens.[306] In accordance with his distinction of physical and spiritual disease, he applauded his own physician for being not only an expert in the profession but for taking "thought also of the correction of spiritual infirmities."[307] Basil considered it a duty of Christian communities to care for the sick. As Gregory of Nazianzus reports,

> "His bodily weakness and his care of the sick made medicine, the fruit of philosophy and industry, a necessity for him. From such a beginning he advanced to mastery of this art, and not only of the branches that deal with the visible and what is immediately apparent, but also of those which deal with principles and theory."[308]

Basil saw diseases as having their cause in nature. Yet God may use them as a means of exhortation of faith: he conceived of interplay between nature and God, yet not nature and demons or evil spirits. He distinguished physical and spiritual disease and health. Whilst recommending medicine for the cure of physical diseases, he viewed health of the soul as being of high importance for overall well-being.

---

302 Quasten, *Patrology III*, 203.
303 Ibid., 204.
304 Ibid.
305 Miller, *Birth of the Hospital*, 87.
306 Gregory of Nazianzus, *On St. Basil*, 23.
307 Basil the Great, *Letter 189*.
308 Gregory of Nazianzus, *On St. Basil*, 23.

In his recognition of the body of medicine and of disease as *of the body* Basil relied heavily on Origen's *Contra Celsum*. However, he went beyond Origen where he recommends medicine for all humans, not only "men of inferior faith" as Origen put it. Medicine is one of God's gifts to humanity and reflects God's will for human salvation. Humans should call in the doctor, but not leave off hoping in God.

Basil's recognition of medicine invited him to reflect on medical practice from the perspective of the good life. Jesus' example in the stories of the New Testament led Basil to a view of *good* medical practice as an act of *charity*: it needs to involve not only *curing* but above all *caring* for all humans, above all those in need (the poor, sick, hungry). Basil's institution outside of the gates of Caesarea allowed him to put this claim to the test.

The linking of cure and care *via* charity persisted beyond Basil's lifetime. Historians of medicine acknowledge *charity* as being at the root of Western medical care.[309] Here, I have been informed by, and will draw on, the general work of historian of medicine Roy Porter, as well as Timothy Miller and Gerhard Harig's writings which focus particularly on the birth of the hospital in late Antiquity and the Byzantine period.

I look at Basil's ethical rules, the *Long Rules*, a synopsis of lectures on the religious life written initially for his community of monks, but also more generally applicable to the ecclesial community outside the walls of the monastery. The focus is on question 55, which deals with the issue of recourse to medicine in case of illness, and is the longest in the collection. Analysing question 55 allows us to see not only Basil's overall position on physical illness, health, and medical healing but moreover his ethical method and principles of decision making. For purposes largely of illustration and contextualisation, I also refer to the writings of Basil's close friend and fellow theologian Gregory of Nazianzus such as *On His Brother, St. Caesarius* and *On St. Basil the Great, Bishop of Caesarea*. Since few handbooks on Patrology speak in explicit terms of the ethical teaching of the Greek Church Fathers[310] (thus, to an extent, fail to acknowledge their writings "as a significant resource for the doing of ethics from within the patristic mind-set and tradition"[311]) the following engages mainly with the primary sources mentioned. However, it is also informed by Stanley S. Hadaka's 1999 *Wholeness of Faith and Life – Orthodox Christian Ethics*, from which the preceding quote has been taken, as well as his 2000 *Health and Medicine in the Eastern Orthodox Tradition*.

---

309 Porter, *Hospitals and Surgery*, 208.
310 See for instance, Quasten (1966); Pelikan (1974), *The Christian Tradition: A History of the Development of Doctrine* and Florovsky (1987), *The Eastern Fathers of the Fourth Century*, Vol. 7 as standard handbooks on Patristic theology where there is little if any treatment of ethics as a theological discipline in the Patristic period.
311 Harakas, *Wholeness of Faith and Life*, 47.

3.5.1 Natural cause and exhortative purpose of disease

Unlike Tatian and Tertullian, Basil the Great saw diseases and death to have "natural causes" – a faulty diet being one of many examples he gives.[312] Diseases are caused by "deficiencies of nature"[313] and of true *human* (as opposed to divine) nature in particular. They are signs of having a natural body.

> "In the case of the Apostle, for instance, in order that he might not seem to exceed the limits of human nature and that no one might think him to possess anything exceptional in his nature [...] he calls attention to his prolonged struggle with an infirmity as a means of demonstrating the fact that he is human."[314]

Or as Gregory of Nazianzus remarks about Basil's brother Caesarius, a famous physician,

> "Although he survived the earthquake, he was not immune to disease, for he was human. His escape was peculiar to himself, his death was common to others; the former was a sign of his piety, the later of his nature."[315]

Diseases as natural deficiencies are often related to the Fall, and may be intended by God as punishment for human sin, Basil says.

> "Not *all* sickness for whose treatment we observe medicine to be occasionally beneficial arise from natural cause, whether from faulty diet or from any other physical origin. Illness is often a punishment for sin."[316]

Before Adam's and Eve's disobedience in the Garden, humans were immune to diseases, Basil says.[317] Only afterwards are

> "We [...] commanded to return to the earth whence we had been taken and (are) united with the pain-ridden flesh doomed to destruction because of sin and, for the same reason, also subject to disease."[318]

Yet where Basil understands diseases as forms of divine punishment, he also has in mind the beneficial nature of such punishment: "Illness is often a punishment for sin, imposed for our conversion."[319] Diseases can be willed by God as trial of faith and might lead to spiritual growth. Basil in *The Long Rules*: "Very often, also, the diseases which we contracted were for our correction and the painful remedies we were obliged to submit to formed part of the instruction."[320] Or in still more explicit terms when he talks about the educational nature of such trials, "God places those who are able to endure tribulation even unto death before the

---

312 Basil the Great, *The Long Rules*, 55.
313 Ibid.
314 Ibid.
315 Gregory of Nazianzus, *On Caesarius*, 16.
316 Basil the Great, *The Long Rules*, 55.
317 Ibid.
318 Ibid.
319 Ibid.
320 Ibid.

weak as their model."[321] In this sense, like Tertullian, Basil thought medical healing might serve as a metaphor for care *and* cure provided by God for the soul:

> "The very transformation of the body from sickness to health should be an incentive to us not
> to despair of the soul, as if it had no power to be restored again through penance from its sin-
> ful state to its proper integrity."[322]

However, unlike Tertullian and Tatian, according to Basil, God acts directly
through and in nature, not indirectly *via* demons and evil spirits. God's means for
bringing about disease is the transformation of bodily nature into a state of defect
which then makes it "susceptible to various hurts, some attacking from without
and some from within by reason of the food we eat."[323]

Basil deals with physical rather than spiritual disease in the first instance. Yet
he refers to the two kinds of disease throughout the *Long Rules*. Sins of the soul,
he says, need to be amended by "assiduous prayer, prolonged penance, and the
severe disciplinary treatment which reason may advise as adequate for the
cure."[324] Similarly, "In caring for our souls we must heal them by accepting the
cut of the reproachful word and the bitter medicine of penalties."[325] Trust in God
must rule out any misplaced views of the physician as saviour; yet at the same
time the art of medicine should be employed. As Basil summarises in the *Long
Rules*, "We call in the doctor but we do not leave off hoping in God."[326] Such
hope and trust in God protects the patient from idolatry, and the physician from
false pride. It also underlines that hope is never exhausted in the case of medical
failure – it may be lost as far as the illness is concerned but not in terms of one's
relationship with God.

3.5.2 Science and art of medicine in the context of salvation

In his reflection on medicine Basil relied heavily on Origen,[327] an Alexandrian
Father, who approved of it as "beneficial and essential to mankind."[328] Origen
"presented an impressive defence of both the use of medicine and the physician's
craft"[329] whilst at the same time conceiving of a link of demons and disease. To
allow for a clearer understanding of this particular background of Basil's thought,
I will sketch out first Origen's position on medicine before looking secondly at
Basil's own account of medical knowledge and practice.

---

321 Basil the Great, *The Long Rules*, 55.
322 Ibid.
323 Ibid.
324 Ibid.
325 Ibid.
326 Ibid.
327 Miller, *Birth of the Hospital*, 55.
328 Origen, *Contra Celsum*, III:12.
329 Miller, *Birth of the Hospital*, 54.

Origen dealt with questions of disease and medicine in *Contra Celsum* (245–250). For him, diseases of the body were appointed as trials of the soul.[330] Whilst he does not detail further causes of disease, Origen acknowledges – like Tatian and Tertullian – the existence of demon-related disease, which requires exorcism: "When the formula 'in the name of Jesus' is pronounced by true believers, it has healed not a few people from diseases and demonic possession and other distresses."[331] However, demons can cause but not cure illness.[332] The invocation of demons "for the sake of bodily health and love of the body"[333] is a sign of distrust in God. Like Tatian, Origen sought to establish God as only master *and* healer of life. Yet against Tatian (and this is where Basil followed him), he held that faith and trust in God did not rule out the recourse to the art of medicine. Origen recommended, "A man ought to use medical means to heal his body *if he aims to live in the simple and ordinary way.*"[334]

The second half of the sentence marks the difference between Origen and Basil. For Origen, medicine is a tool of healing for humans of *inferior* faith. To place one's trust in God's healing powers *alone* is a gift not given to everyone. It pertains to the superior way of life, which is for Origen the way of the monk or the monastic community. "If man wishes to live in a way superior to that of the multitude, he should do this by devotion to the supreme God and by praying to Him."[335]

Basil followed Origen's affirmation of grace "as evident in the healing power of medicine and the skill of its practitioners."[336] And like Origen, Basil considered it a mistake to make medicine "wholly accountable for our state of health or illness"[337] and to place one's hope in the doctor alone. Whilst avoiding a blanket rejection or unqualified recognition of medicine, he developed Origen's view further in that he recommends medicine to all humans and Christians, not only the 'inferior Christians' outside of monastic communities.

In *The Long Rules* under the heading "whether recourse to the medical art is in keeping with the practice of piety"[338] (a question which expresses a certain suspicion that the use of medicine might imply a lack of faith), Basil accounted for reasons for a positive recognition of medical knowledge and therapies. Natural knowledge, he said, depends in its worth and usefulness on the will of the user:

> "We know that neither fire nor food nor iron nor any other element is in itself either very useful or very harmful, but that all depends on the will of the user. Even from certain reptiles we have at times compounded salutary medicines. So also from the pagans we have received

---

330 Origen, *Contra Celsum*, VIII:56.
331 Ibid., VIII:58.
332 Ibid., VIII:60.
333 Ibid., VIII:61.
334 Ibid., VIII:60 (my italics).
335 Ibid., VIII:60.
336 Risse, *Mending Bodies*, 77.
337 Basil the Great, *The Long Rules*, 55.
338 Ibid.

principles of inquiry and speculation, while we have rejected what ever leads to demons and error and the abyss of perdition."[339]

Further, *all* human arts, hence also the medical art, are divine institutions for the benefit of humanity. Even where medicine is perhaps badly practised or sinfully utilised, humans ought not to avoid the good that medicine is able to offer. Basil places the question of the propriety of using the medical arts or not within the context of theological concepts and teachings, namely the doctrine of God as Creator who shows providential care for his creation both as a whole, and for the human creature in particular. In Basil's words,

> "Each of these arts is God's gift to us remedying the deficiencies of nature, as for example, agriculture, since the produce which the earth bears of itself would not suffice to provide for our needs; the art of weaving, since the use of clothing is necessary for decency's sake and for protection from the wind; and similarly the art of building. The same is true also for the medical art. In as much as our body is susceptible to various hurts, some attacking from without and some from within by reason of the food we eat, and since the body suffers affliction from both excess and deficiency, the medical art has been vouchsafed us by God, who directs our whole life, as a model for the cure of the soul, to guide us in the removal of what is superfluous and in the addition of what is lacking."[340]

Four aspects of this statement are worth further reflection. First, in addressing monks, Basil speaks to men whom Origen considered "superior Christians" and whom he recommended *not* to employ medicine. Basil, however, does not conceive of a hierarchy of higher and lower Christians; instead he insists, as Peter Brown remarks, that *every* baptised Christian "was under an obligation to become, day by day, a little more like his [Basil's] own austere idea of a monk."[341] For Basil, the idea of life in monastic-like brotherhoods sharing a life of poverty and charity reflects Christian praxis. *All* baptised Christians should strive for a life in poverty and charity, thus moving, to use Origen's terms, from lower to higher Christians. And since medicine as the art of caring for the sick belongs to the praxis of charity, all Christians should not hesitate to refer to its knowledge. Indeed, as will be further explored below, the use of medicine is not only in accordance with, but also serves the goal of piety.

Secondly, Basil speaks of medical practise in classical Galenic terms, which shows his acceptance of natural, medical knowledge and practice. The causes of diseases are either excess or deficiency, Basil says, so that removal or addition of substances will cure them. "In the case of the flesh it is essential to eliminate foreign elements and add whatever is wanting."[342] Similarly, Galen described doctors as overseers and care-takers of bodies, who "recognise what substance a body is lacking, and how much of this substance" and "cure the loss immediately by introducing the same amount of substance."[343] Basil also mentions concrete ex-

---

339 Gregory of Nazianzus, *On St. Basil*, 11.
340 Basil the Great, *The Long Rules*, 55.
341 Brown, *Body and Society*, 291. Cf. on the importance of community life, Basil, *The Long Rules*, 7.
342 Basil the Great, *The Long Rules*, 55.
343 Galen, *To Thrasyboulos*, 69.

amples of ancient medical practice, when he says, "in using the medical art we submit to cutting, burning, and the taking of bitter medicines."[344] Later he adds abstinence from food as therapeutic measure, which was a common treatment in Galenic medicine.[345]

Thirdly, and perhaps most importantly, the art of medicine is given to humans by God "to relieve the sick"[346] just like fruits and water can be found in nature for the relief of hunger and thirst. Medicine's natural tools express God's care for humanity. Herbal remedies show God's providential care present in nature (which is neither totally corrupted nor essentially intact, according to Basil).

> "The herbs which are the specifics for each malady do not grow out of the earth sponta-
> neously; it is evidently the will of the Creator that they should be brought forth out of the soil
> to serve our need. Therefore the obtaining of that natural virtue which is in the roots and
> flowers, leaves, fruits, and juices, or in such metals or products of the sea as are found espe-
> cially suitable for bodily health, is to be viewed in the same way as the procuring of food and
> drink."[347]

Whilst Basil does not reject natural medicine, his answer to question 55 shows that his basic presupposition is derived from his theological understanding of God as Creator, who shows providential care to his creation, and in particular to the human creature. Further, God's care present in the art of medicine and the gifts of nature, which ought to be used by humans in the service of healing, indicates "the synergy between what might be called the common (non-redemptive) grace of God and the human component in the elementary response to the consequences of the fallen condition of humanity."[348]

Fourthly, medicine provides an analogy for the healing of the soul. It is "a parallel to the care given the soul."[349] In yet stronger words, "It is an example for the *proper* care of the soul."[350] It is an art that serves as analogy for God's healing of the soul. The use of medicine as analogy to spiritual restoration and of Christ as the *archiatros*, the highest physician, administering the medicine of his word to those sick in souls, is a recurrent motive in the *Long Rules* as well as in Eastern Christian literature and Byzantine iconic art. The *Christos medicus* metaphor is also a practical expression of the Chalcedonies teaching regarding the incarnation, which affirms the intimate relationship of human and divine, natural and spiritual, in the one person Jesus Christ while maintaining the difference between the divine and the created overall.

Despite the emphasis on the spiritual life, it is, however, necessary to learn how to use the gift of medicine *properly* so that human usage does not destroy the intentions of the giver.[351] Humans ought not commit outrage against God by put-

---

344 Basil the Great, *The Long Rules*, 55.
345 Ibid.
346 Ibid.
347 Ibid.
348 Harakas, *Wholeness of Faith and Life*, 84.
349 Basil the Great, *The Long Rules*, 55.
350 Ibid (my italics).
351 Ibid.

ting his gift to bad use. Basil's view calls for judgement: what, then, is a "proper way" of using medicine? When is medicine *good* medical practice in accordance with the goodness of its giver? Basil's recognition of medicine allows him to reflect on the way in which medicine should be done "properly": humans should focus on the spiritual dimension of existence,[352] and good medical practice is bound up with the good life of which the New Testament gives testimony.

3.5.3 The good life, medical care, and the first hospital

In search for the good life, young Basil was drawn to solitaries and monastic communities. However, when he saw the monks of Egypt, Palestine and Syria, he was not only amazed by their ascetic heroics but "struck too by their failure to carry out the corporeal works of mercy"[353] and by their failure of *koinonia*, of community, in which service for the world is practised. It was here that Basil was confronted with the question of the appropriate relationship of *praxis* and *theoria*.

Theoria, that is teaching and preaching, praying and worshipping, always takes place within an ecclesial community. In being *theoria* within a community, it not only sustains human knowledge of God's presence but also provides humans with a community that is able to sustain human presence to others in pain. Drawing on his reading of the scriptures, Basil understood that Christ expected his followers *to be present* – that is, to feed the hungry, clothe the naked and care for the sick. This means, to carry out practical works of charity and *philanthropeia*. "Prayer and psalmody" are no excuses "for neglecting their work, it is necessary to bear in mind that for certain other tasks a particular time is allotted."[354]

In the end, Basil the Great turned his back on a form of ascetic life that ignored praxis: for the good life, it is necessary to incorporate both *theoria* and *praxis*, both prayer and works of mercy, and to do this in a community of people, he concluded. The phrase "If you live alone, whose feet will you wash?" pointedly highlights the distinctions between solitude and collective service[355] as well as between the active life of *praxis* (deeds of charity in and for the community) and the life of *theoria* (worship, prayer within or outwit a community).

Basil starts his instruction for monks with an exposition of the commandment of love of God and one's neighbour, thus explaining its predominance for both *theoria* and *praxis* in the Christian life.[356] Charity belongs to the very nature of human beings. It is a seed in everyone, planted in anticipation of the Lord's requiring fruits of charity, Basil says. Charitable acts are a means of recognising Christ's disciples and are ultimately transferred to Jesus Christ Himself.[357]

---

352 Harakas, *Wholeness of Faith and Life,* 86.
353 Miller, *Birth of the Hospital*, 119.
354 Basil the Great, *The Long Rules*, 37.
355 Risse, *Mending Bodies*, 76/Basil, *The Long Rules*, 7.
356 Basil the Great, *The Long Rules*, 1.
357 Mt. 25:40, Cf. Basil the Great, *The Long Rules*, 3/*The Morals*, Rule 3.

Whilst charity points to the importance of care in Basil's approach to medicine, his second concern regarding the good life, which is the need for a community of people, needs to be looked at a bit further. Where somebody is all by himself, he will always fail to act out one of the many dimensions of charity.[358]

> "For example, when he is visiting the sick, he cannot show hospitality to the stranger and, in the imparting and sharing of necessities [...] he is prevented from giving zealous attention to other tasks. As a result, the greatest commandment and the one especially conducive to salvation is not observed, since the hungry are not fed nor the naked clothed."[359]

A monastic community with a whole range of charitable institutions would best serve the requirements of the good life which takes seriously the example Christ gave, Basil thought, and founded in 370 a philanthropic institution, a *ptochotropeion*[360] outside the gates of Caesarea. Gregory of Nazianzus refers to this institution as 'the new city'. He says,

> "Go forth a little from this city and behold the new city, the storehouse of piety, the common treasury of the wealthy where superfluous riches, sometimes even necessities, thanks to the exhortations of Basil are laid up, unexposed to the moths and no source of joy for the thief, escaping the assault of envy and the corruption of time."[361]

Gregory's evocation of Basil's "new city" was not simply fourth century rhetoric but represented a new Christian self-understanding, which combined the Hellenistic call to social and political leadership based on social class status with the call to be disciples of Christ through practical action as leaders in the church community. Indeed, "new city" seems appropriate considering the enormous cluster of various institutions and facilities, in which care was provided under the supervision of one single superior.[362] The "new city" was explicitly set up so that Christian charity could be put into practice. Hence, it was conceived as a new *Christian* city that now existed outside the old secular town of Caesarea. Basil's foundation was for Gregory of Nazianzus "the most wonderful achievement of all, the short road to salvation and the easiest ascent to heaven."[363] As Basil says in *Letter 94*, it was "a source of pride to the governor since words of praise redound upon him."

For Basil himself "the new city" was the epitome of true Christian life in so far as it enabled humans to follow the highest commandment and live in discipleship to Jesus Christ. This new city was founded as a city *in* and *for* the world not as a supposedly *heavenly* sphere detached from, or distant to it.

The care of the sick played a crucial role. Gregory of Nazianzus in his funeral sermon does not refer explicitly to the care of poor people or strangers but says, "There, sickness is endured with equanimity, calamity is a blessing, and sympathy is put to the test."[364] The service of the sick is accounted for as deep expression of

---

358 Basil the Great, *The Long Rules*, 7.
359 Ibid.
360 *Ptochos* means 'poor', *trepho* means 'to nourish', *ptochotropheion* in the literal sense designates a house to shelter and feed the destitute.
361 Gregory of Nazianzus, *On St. Basil*, 63.
362 Miller, *Birth of the Hospital*, 87.
363 Gregory of Nazianzus, *On St. Basil*, 63.
364 Ibid.

sympathy, charity, and love of humanity (*philanthropeia*), an embodiment of the Christian calling to become God-like. "God was above all *philanthropos*, 'one who loves humanity'."[365] Reportedly, Basil took the care for the sick upon himself in the *ptochotropeion*. "Others had their cooks and rich tables and enchanting refinements of cuisine, and elegant carriages, and soft flowing garments", Gregory says; "Basil had his sick, and the dressing of their wounds, and the imitation of Christ, cleansing leprosy not by word but in deed."[366]

A hospital, in which both cure and care took place, was part of the cluster of different institutions. It included most definitely physicians as part of its staff.[367] The *Basileias* is considered the first hospital in Western civilisation whereby hospital is understood as an establishment for the cure *and* care of the sick or wounded regardless of their profession, economic and social class, sex, age and race etc.[368] Indeed, no traces were found of hospitals before Basil's institution in Caesarea. The Roman *valetudinarian*, which provided treatment and care, were designed only to serve restricted groups of people, army personnel in the first place. The Greek *asclepiad* did neither provide accommodation nor food nor other forms of nursing care; Greek *atria* or doctor's surgeries equally had no place of accommodation and care for the sick.[369]

As Timothy Miller remarked,

> "The Orthodox Christians of the East not only accepted Greek medicine: they moved it to a central place in their theological system. [...] They came to see the medical profession as a symbol of charity in action, the cornerstone of Christian morality."[370]

And he continued that Basil's high estimation of medicine and its relation to Christian morality helped to bring into existence the hospitals as first institutions of charity.

The significance of care in the institutionalised public sense of the *Basileias* as well as in a more individual way is brought out most forcefully by Gregory of Nazianzus in the above mentioned sermon 14 titled *Love of the Poor*. Whilst also looking at social exclusion and poverty more generally, the sermon largely deals with the misery of lepers, i.e. those who are excluded society due to the visible effects leprosy had on their skin and the perceived risk of contagion. The image of the leper's body as Christ's body is present throughout the sermon.

The oration was written during 369–371, most likely as an appeal for support for Basil's efforts in providing public care for the sick (mainly lepers) and poor, though there is no direct evidence in the sermon of Basil's social activities. It is written as a homiletic appeal to moral action, to individual participation in assisting the poor.

---

365 Harakas, *Health in the Orthodox Tradition*, 75.
366 Gregory of Nazianzus, *On St. Basil*, 63.
367 Basil, *Letter 94*.
368 Miller, *Birth of the Hospital*, 30–39.
369 Cf. Miller, *Birth of the Hospital*, 30–39; Risse, *Mending Bodies*, 56 ff.
370 Miller, *Birth of the Hospital*, 61.

The redemptive nature of the "love of humanity" is what Nazianzus sets out to examine. He begins by a discussion of which virtue is supreme and finds that love of the poor and compassion and sympathy is the most excellent form of Christian charity. Whilst he wrote it partly in a spiritualising mode where physical affliction (here: leprosy) is used as metaphor for the illness of the soul such as debauchery, above all he addresses physical disfigurement, which afflicts people involuntarily. He talks about the social exclusion disfigurement is accompanied with. He explains that the kindness and compassion we show towards our brothers and sisters in misery "is the single way towards the salvation both of our bodies and of our souls." He invites his audience to come into physical contact with the lepers, for touch – medically contagious it was believed to be – is theologically salvific: it will effect spiritual healing for those who are physically well.

Two points are interesting in this context: like Gregory of Nyssa before him, Gregory Nazianzus sees lepers (and the poor) as belonging to humanity. They are humans like us; they are our *kin*, our brothers and sisters, both literally and metaphorically.

Secondly, he sees them in their relationship to the divine, so that the love we show to them as our kin is love shown to Christ:

> "Brothers and sisters, we must care for what is part of our nature and shares in our slavery. [...] And we must, each of us, care no less for our neighbours' bodies than our own, the bodies both of those who are healthy and of those who are consumed by this disease. 'For we are all one in the Lord, whether rich or poor, whether slave or free, whether in good health of body or in bad; and there is one head of all, from whom all things proceed: Christ'."[371]

Whilst both the two Gregories and Basil focus on similar ideas (common humanity, the superiority of actions over words, and of charity as the highest command) of the three writings it is Gregory of Nazianzus whose sermon on the poor most explicitly recommends the philanthropic care for the disfigured as action of love, the greatest of all virtues. He emphasises a view of the poor and disfigured as incarnation of Christ – hence, he says, our attitude towards them reflects our attitude to Christ. To quote the passage in full,

> "Do you think that kindness to others is not a necessity for you, but a matter of choice? That it is not a law, but simply an exhortation? [...] Let us take care of Christ while there is still time; let us minister to Christ's needs, let us give Christ nourishment, let us clothe Christ, let us gather Christ in, let us show Christ honour [...] Let us give this gift to him through the needy, who today are cast down on the ground, so that when we all are released from this place, they may receive is into the eternal tabernacle, in Christ himself, who is our Lord."[372]

3.5.4 Concluding remarks

> "In general [the Church Fathers] regarded physical health as a relative good, but not an end in itself and by no means essential to spiritual health, which they considered more important. Yet most maintained that the body was to be reasonably cared for because God had provided

---

371 Gregory, *Oration* 14, 8.
372 Ibid., 39–40.

the means for its care. Health was a blessing from God, but God sometimes used poor health as a spiritual discipline."[373]

Against a standard medical history which asserts that rational medicine did not fare well in Byzantium and the first Christian millennium more generally, it has been shown that both Tertullian and Basil the Great disapproved of certain of their fellows who accepted death all to readily and did not seek help through medicine. Despite a markedly different view of the relationship of theological, philosophical, and medical claims, they both considered an outright rejection of medicine as rejection of God's good intentions for humankind. In Basil's words, medical knowledge and treatment have advantages for both body and soul[374] so that "to reject entirely the benefits to be derived from this art is the sign of a pettish nature."[375]

Yet in contrast to his Latin predecessor Tertullian, and above all Tatian, Basil was keen to engage with philosophy. Philosophical principles of inquiry and speculation can be accepted if used in the right way,[376] which is in following the commandment of love of God and the neighbour. If in its practice naturalist medicine is *mimesis Christi* and serves charity within the community, it is not to be rejected. Rather, where it exemplifies the central Christian virtue of loving care it must pertain to the good life: it is *a good* in being God's gift to humanity, and it is *one of the highest goods* of the Christian life, for it is the epitome of charity in action.[377] From the evidence of the *Basileias* one can conclude that Basil not only took on board secular medicine as a necessary and competent means of healing, but specifically intended to place it in the centre of his theological system and the Christian life in community in general.

This allowed him to introduce Christian morality into medical practice. The manner in which medical healing should be performed is guided by the commandment of twofold love, which posits God as the highest value, thus limiting the value of medicine. Spiritual health and spiritual healing are to be valued higher. Yet, as Harakas points out,

> "This, of course, does not mean that whenever there is a reasonable hope that therapeutic methods might succeed treatment should not be vigorously pursued. Basil's view allows for judgment and permits the cessation of treatments that are of improbable effectiveness. For Basil, however, this is not abandonment, but a focus on the spiritual dimensions of human life and existence."[378]

For Basil, ethical teaching both in general and in the medical context in particular is derived from theological belief, not philosophical inquiry. Implicated in his answer to question 55 is a hierarchy of values – the relationship with God in the first instance followed by spiritual goodness, which is at all times bound up with the good of the body. The primacy of God's relationship with humans, and of spiritual goodness over against bodily goodness, should guide decision-making: it

---

373 Amundsen, "Early Christian Tradition", 59.
374 Basil the Great, *The Long Rules*, 55.
375 Ibid.
376 Gregory of Nazianzus, *On St. Basil*, 11.
377 Miller, *Birth of the Hospital*, 56.
378 Harakas, *Wholeness of Faith and Life*, 86.

provides humans with an understanding of the *telos* of their actions (namely the "practice of piety" and the spiritual fulfilment of life) and a judgement on the means employed to achieve such *tells*. Most importantly, perhaps, for Basil such decision-making is understood as a process which happens within the ecclesial community, not as personal or individual deciding.

Basil emphasised the importance for human fulfilment and happiness of knowing the command of charity, which posits God as the highest value, and involves compassionate cure and care for the other, thus emphasising "the sense of human corporations and ecclesial unity."[379] He reminded his readers *that* one needs to be present to the sick, and to seek to cure him or her, without however reflecting what the personal implications of this presence might be. Whilst Basil's emphasis throughout is on the physical, spiritual and socio-*communal* dimension of human existence, it remains unclear (for his anthropology is not spelled out) whether personal and individual aspects of human life are also included in this view.

Going back to the initial question of the relationship of medicine and Christianity, for early Christian writers such as Tatian at the one end, and Basil at the other end of the spectrum, rational medicine was distinguished from spiritual healing. For some it was subsumed under religion. For others, it would not be sharply divided from spiritual healing. For the Greek Fathers in particular Harakas emphasises,

> "In their writings some of the Byzantine fathers emphasised the discontinuity between faith and non-revelatory knowledge, asserting the transcendence of faith, while others focused on the communion and continuity of faith and worldly knowledge. Nevertheless, in general Orthodox Christians in Byzantium held faith-truths and scientific-truths together in a single perspective."[380]

Certainly, Basil's philanthropic institution in Caesarea is the strongest evidence of such a wholesome and cooperative relationship between the Orthodox Christian tradition and rational medicine.

Against the background of the above, Nutton's thesis of medicine and Christianity as two independent spheres of action is questionable. Von Harnack, on the other hand, in claiming Christianity to be a "medical religion" rightly emphasised the intrinsic link between Christian revelation and medical healing, which has been affirmed in more recent work on Byzantine and Western approaches to medicine.[381] Von Harnack, however, fell short of showing medicine's specific scope which can be derived from a Christian understanding of human life. Being concerned with establishing both historically and theologically the relationship of medicine and Christianity, von Harnack did not give attention to the health of the soul or human morality, thus restricting Christianity's concern with health and healing to the body. Also, he did not take into consideration the contributions Au-

---

379 Harakas, *Wholeness of Faith and Life*, 89.
380 Harakas, *Health in the Orthodox Tradition*, 71.
381 See for instance John Scarborough (ed.): *Symposium on Byzantine Medicine*, Dumbarton Oaks Papers 38 (Washington, 1985).

gustine made for our understanding of humans in body and soul, and what this can tell us for the practice of medicine, the human will to cure, the understanding we have of health, and the health of the human soul.

To address these questions, I turn to St. Augustine (354–430), the Church Father who more than any other shaped Christian theology and anthropology in the light of the command of love. Augustine's coherent anthropology is an influential Christian reflection, developed in contemplating, and drawing from Scripture, in particular the book of Genesis. Such theological reflection on life which integrates the natural, personal, and social against the background of the doctrines of incarnation and resurrection provides the foundation for Augustine's view of health and disease as states of life, and for his attitude towards medicine as a tool given by God for the benefit of humanity.

4. CONCEPTUALISING HEALTH (2): AUGUSTINE ON HEALTH AND HEALING

Motivated by the normative function of health and the fragmentary approaches the contemporary philosophical debate revealed, this study reflects with early Christian writers and philosophers on the anthropological requirements for a coherent conceptual framework of health and medical healing. The thesis is that such a framework needs to include the interplay of the natural-bodily, socio-personal, and moral-spiritual dimension of human life, which are implicated in the state of health, and therefore in the clinical encounter, in clinically oriented medical research, and in health care policy making.

Galen of Pergamon started from a unified vision of human life in body and soul. And in allowing for the corrective influence of reason on human behaviour, Galen moved beyond a purely functional account of body and soul, and hence, of health and of clinical practice. His analysis of the union of body and soul, and of human improvement as the context for health considerations, was taken further by looking at three early Christian writers who explored health and medical healing within these parameters (that is, of the union of body/soul on the one hand, and improvement/full well-being on the other hand). Structurally not unlike Galen, early Christian writers sought to account for the patient as a person in the union of body and soul. Yet unlike Galen, they looked at the body-soul union not from the body, but from God's revelation in Christ, and did not understand this union *functionally* but *hierarchically,* the soul being above the body and guiding its actions. Whilst they all maintained that the body was to be cared for, the interplay of nature, the supernatural (demons) and spiritual (divine) was assessed differently and led to an attitude towards medical healing ranging from rejection, to tentative recognition, to acknowledgment as the epitome of charity. Due to their theological perspective on nature and human mortality, they were highly sceptical as regards any lasting and real improvement through natural knowledge – not only of the human character or the soul but also of the body. On the basis of such scepticism boundaries may be set up that prevent a mediatisation of life.

Anthropology is the area in which "Augustine's mind primarily works."[382] In his anthropology, Augustine is most original. Here, he achieves a high degree of coherence in that he integrates the natural, personal, social and spiritual dimensions of existence on the basis of the doctrines of creation, incarnation and resurrection.

Exploring Augustine's anthropology in its relevance for health and healing, I proceed from universals to particulars (that is, from the creation of the world to the creation of humans) and from the past to the present to the future life (that is, from human life before and after the Fall to the future life *post resurrectionem*).

I start with a brief introduction on Augustine's view on creation and the Creator, which explains human life as both given and in *a priori* relationship with its Creator. Created existence according to God's word is *good* and *ordered*. Created bodies exist in a hierarchical order of relationships, which originates in the relational love of the Trinitarian God.[383] This irrevocably attributes value to the whole that is creation and to all its parts: whatever *is*, also and always is *good*.

Human existence is material and bodily, yet it is never the life of the body only. The body-soul union is central to Augustine's anthropology. Together with the incarnation, Christ's resurrection affirms the goodness of the body. In the resurrection, the body is taken up into eternity where it remains the very same, particular body (*my* body or *your* body). Augustine shows that both the incarnation and resurrection are the foundation of the Christian understanding of the intrinsic and inalienable goodness of the human body. The body's value needs to be born in mind especially in the context of the physical evil of disease.

Whilst recognising the goodness of the body, Augustine holds that the soul is the creature's superior part. The soul not only animates, but also dominates the body. It is the site of the image of God in humans. I will look closely at three particular aspects of Augustine's interpretation of the *imago*, namely, the relational, dynamic, proleptic aspects. The *imago* constitutes the intrinsically *personal* dimension of human life (a human being is the particular *you* in God's loving address) as well as its *social* dimension, that is, its intrinsic direction to the other, who is also addressed as *you*.[384] This love grounds an attitude towards the other and oneself that is at all times *qualified* through creation, incarnation and redemption.

My inquiry into Augustine's view of the soul in the context of the image of God includes looking at his interpretation of the Fall: due to the Fall, the image of God's love in humans is "discoloured", Augustine says. It is in need of renewal or restoration. This restoration is brought to humans in Christ and mediated by the Spirit; it means that the soul is in a process of renewal, of moving closer to God's love, and ultimately to the eschatological fullness of love and life.

Though Augustine resolutely defended the goodness of matter, he was also painfully aware of the deficiencies of nature which humans experience most acutely in bodily illness and in the encounter with death. And he understood *evil* in nature as God's punishment for the freely chosen disobedience in the Garden. Such punishment for Augustine is just and inherited. At the same time, it can be earned through individual acts of disobedience. Augustine did not look for a purely rationalistic solution to the problem of evil in the world, to which the question of causes of disease belongs. Bodily evil such as disease functions as an exhortation to the conversion of people's hearts to God's love, and is thus linked

---

383 Augustine, *City of God*, XI/10.
384 Augustine, *Trinity*, VIII/10.

with the human soul. God's salvific love revealed in Christ is the primary context in which Augustine reflected on disease, health, and (medical) healing.

Bodily health is a gift of grace which belongs to the history of human salvation. It reflects God's end for humanity: happiness, joy, and well-being. Augustine saw medicine as one possible means of healing; it is God's mercy and grace working in the medical profession. God is also known to have healed in the sacrament of baptism and in response to prayer.

Like Tertullian, Augustine distinguished disease and health of body and soul. Illness of the soul (the discolouring of the *imago*) is a result of humanity's separation from God's love after the Fall. This separation leads to love of self, instead of love of God, and to behaviour such as lust, envy or greed. The full restoration of the *imago* (hence, of the creature's relationship to God, self, and the other) is not a sudden and immediate event. It is a gradual process, which takes place during one's lifetime and will be completed in the escheating. Healing of the soul needs to be striven for first, in remitting the cause in baptism, and second, in orienting one's *self* to the love of God and meeting others on this basis. The soul's health is valued higher than all bodily health: it leads the human creature as a whole (that is, in its union of body and soul) to the fullness of love in the escheating.

Covering Augustine's life-time from his conversion almost up to his death, the selection of writings dealt with in the following not only contain his main thoughts on human life but attempt to do justice to the chronological development of his thinking. Augustine was a systematic thinker whose thought developed through dialogue with Scriptures, but he wrote as a bishop responding to ecclesial and moral issues, at times also with religion-political ends in mind. His thought responded to, was provoked by, and developed in the course of, the ecclesial controversies he was involved in as a Catholic bishop: for example, those between Catholics and Manichees, Donatists or Pelagians. Where required, as well as time and space permitting, the influence of Augustine's adversaries will also be taken into consideration.

Due to the vast amount of Augustine's writings the following exposition refers to a selection of main pieces of work. Beside one of his earliest works, *The Catholic and the Manichean Way of Life* (written in 387/8 shortly after his conversion to Christianity), the following is based upon *The Confessions* (397–401), *The Trinity* (399–422/426), *The Expositions of the Psalms* (392–422), *The Literal Interpretation of Genesis* (completed 416) and *The City of God* (413–427).

4.1 CREATION AND CREATOR

In exploring *creation*, Augustine was not interested in an inquiry into the different scientific theories of his times about the process (or processes) thought to have caused the universe. He speaks about creation as the beginning of existence and speaks about it in the imagined and theological sense. According to this tradition, the universe, which includes all temporal things in heaven and on earth, temporal human life, animals, plants and inanimate objects, *is* because God gratuitously willed it to *be*. In the fallen world, that is the concrete world humans know, God reaffirms his love as both the basis of, and reason for his authorship of (and authority over) creation.

This section starts with Augustine on the nature of God, the Creator, followed by an exposition of God's creation of the world through his word and *ex nihilo*.

I look at Augustine's understanding of the order of created existence derived from the order within the tri-personal God and his understanding of the intrinsic and inalienable goodness of created matter.

Looking at creation and the Creator allows me to explicate how human life is a gift, placed in relationship to God, the life-giver. This view is foundational for Augustine's later dealing with health, disease, death, and medicine. Throughout, other strands of his doctrine of creation will be taken up such as *creation-ex-nihilo* (see Augustine's view of the Fall, disease, and human sinfulness), order of existence (see his understanding of order within the body-soul union, and the hierarchy of health of soul/health of body), and the goodness of matter (see his recognition of the body as good in the face of its susceptibility to disease and death).

Augustine developed his theology of creation in dialogue with, and as a critique of, Platonic and Manichean cosmologies; to do this he drew on, and interpreted, the account of creation provided in the book of Genesis. Against the Manichees, he defended a literal understanding of Genesis; in the rest of his writings on Genesis he insisted on the hermeneutic principle of the existence of a deeper, allegorical meaning.[385] *On Genesis Against the Manichees* (388–390) is Augustine's first interpretation of the Genesis account, followed by *On the Literal Interpretation of Genesis – an Unfinished Book* (393–394), the last three books of *The Confessions* (397–401), *On the Literal Interpretation of Genesis* (completed 416) and book eleven of *The City of God* (419–420).

4.1.1 The Creator

Both the scriptures and the universe disclose the divine authorship of the world. God as cause of all existence is the foundation of Augustine's theology and of his theological anthropology.[386]

With reference to the book of Genesis, Augustine proclaims God as Creator of the world. "That God made the world, we can believe from no one more securely than from God Himself. Where have we heard Him? Nowhere more clearly than in the Holy Scriptures."[387] Even if the voices of the prophets were silent, humans would be able to discern their lives' divine author, since the world

> "Proclaims by a kind of silent testimony of its own, both that it has been created and also that it could not have been made other than by a God ineffable and invisible in greatness."[388]

---

385 Weber, *Genesis contra Manichaeos*, 300.
386 Christian, "Creation", 315.
387 Augustine, *City of God*, XI/4.
388 Augustine, *City of God*, XI/4. Cf. Rom 1.

The scriptures witness to the Creator as the Trinity of Father, Son and Holy Spirit.

> "Where the name of God occurs, I have come to see the Father who made these things; where the 'Beginning' is mentioned, I see the Son by whom he made these things. Believing that my God is Trinity, in accordance with my belief, I searched in God's holy oracles and found your Spirit to be borne above the waters. There is the Trinity, my God – Father and Son and Holy Spirit, Creator of the entire creation."[389]

Hence, it is the *triune* God who is the cause of everything that exists. Yet what or who is this triune God? In Scripture, he has revealed himself to humanity as *being*. He is the "I am he who is" of the Hebrew Bible.[390] He is the "most high, utterly good, utterly powerful, most omnipotent, most merciful and most just."[391] Augustine emphasised the *intrinsic* nature of God as being and goodness: the divine attributes are not qualities attributed to God like the alienable properties ascribed to ordinary worldly things and to people. There is no distinction between *is* and *has* in God. God's attributes *are* his being.[392] They are literally inalienable and *not* something different from what God *is*. They are not different to God –

> "In the way that a vessel is different from its liquid or a body from its colour or the air from its light or heat, or the mind from its wisdom. [...] None of these things is what it has: the vessel is not liquid; the body is not colour; the air is not light or heat; the mind is not wisdom: the vessel may be emptied of the liquid of which it is full; the body may be discoloured; the air may grow dark or cold; the mind become foolish."[393]

So God *is* wisdom, goodness, power, omnipotence, mercy and justice. He can never be deprived of his wisdom, goodness, power, omnipotence, mercy and justice, nor can he be turned or changed into other states or qualities: the qualities he *has* are what he *is*.

4.1.2 Creatio-ex-nihilo

The next question on Augustine's mind concerned the origins of creation. The doctrine of a creation out-of-nothing, *creatio-ex-nihilo*, which by the fourth century had become a standard doctrine of the Church,[394] was the only view of creation as both the visible world and the invisible realm of angels which he thought compatible with the doctrine of God as first cause and absolute goodness.

Where God is seen as wholly goodness, omnipotence and freedom, no sense can be made of a doctrine that portrays God as forming the world according to the constraints of pre-existing formless matter. This is, however, what the Manichees claimed. Augustine argued against Manichean cosmology that no matter could have existed beside God, for "how could you obtain anything you had not made as

---

389 Augustine, *Confessions*, XIII/v/6.
390 Exodus 3:14.
391 Augustine, *Confessions*, I/iv/4.
392 Gilson, *Augustine*, 217.
393 Augustine, *City of God*, XI/10.
394 Knuuttila, "Time and Creation", 103.

a tool for making something? What is it for something to be unless it is because you are?"[395]

If, for instance, God had created the world out of his own substance, Augustine says, one part of his substance – then used as material for the world – would have become finite and changeable: decay and finitude mark all worldly substance. Yet this would contradict God's absolute and eternal, infinite and unchangeable being. Further, it would mean that the world was equal to the Son, who alone is of divine substance, and therefore alone equal to God himself. The Son alone is the perfect image and resemblance of the Father. As Augustine says:

> "You made heaven and earth not of your own self, or it would be equal to your only-begotten Son and therefore to yourself. It cannot possibly be right for anything which is not of you to be equal to you."[396]

Against this background, Augustine concluded,

> "There was nothing apart from you out of which you could make them, God one in three and three in one. [...] You were, the rest was nothing. Out of nothing you made heaven and earth."[397]

God made the world from formless matter, which he created out of nothing; he "made this next-to-nothing out of nothing, and from it you made great things at which the sons of men wonder."[398]

Yet how did he create out-of-nothing? In accordance with the Genesis account Augustine holds that God created the world through the power of his word: "Therefore you spoke and they were made, and by your word you made them."[399] Through the power of the divine command, ontologically *new* things and beings came into existence.

4.1.3 Order of existence

These new beings, which constitute creation and exist through God's word, are in motion; they realise their potentials and grow in order and beauty.[400] All created beings have the inherent power of development, which for Augustine is the potential both of natural development *and* of being acted upon by God.[401] All created things exist in time. Change belongs to temporal existence. Human existence is temporal, mutable, and incomplete; it is *becoming* in the face of God, the eternal, unchanging, and complete. Created existence, then, finds itself in constant motion and subject to change. Yet it is never a wild, unstructured, anarchical floating around of created entities. Created bodies exist within the universe in a specific

395 Augustine, *Confessions*, XI/v/7.
396 Ibid., XII/vii/7.
397 Ibid.
398 Ibid., XII/viii/8.
399 Ibid., XI/v/7.
400 Augustine, *Literal interpretation of Genesis*, 6.14.25–6.18.29/9.17.31–32.
401 Ibid., 6.14.25.

order, the *ordo rerum* or *ordo naturae* – a concept of order which underpins the concept of natural law.[402] In Augustine's words,

> "Those which have life are placed above those which do not have life; and those that have the power of generation, or even of desiring it, are placed above those which lack this capacity. And, among living things, the sentient are placed above those which do not have sensation: animals above trees, for instance. And among the sentient, the intelligent are placed above those which do not have intelligence: men, for example, are above cattle. And among the intelligent, the immortals, such as the angels, are placed above the mortals such as men. These are the gradations which exist in the order of nature."[403]

Augustine's view of the universal order as a hierarchy of relationships "embraces the entire created universe from the lowest level of inanimate being to the immortal angelic spirits, as representing the highest rank among rational essences."[404] The order of nature is divinely instituted order and is harmony and peace.[405] It is to be respected, if good existence is to be preserved.

> "All natures, then, simply because they exist and therefore have a species of their own, a kind of their own, and a certain peace of their own are certainly good. And when they are where they should be according to the order of their nature, they preserve their own being according to the measure in which they have received it."[406]

The order of created existence originates within the Trinity itself, precisely within the relational love of its three persons, "for the Holy Ghost unites the Father and the Son in self-subsistent Love, which is both the Model and Source of all creaturely order and love."[407] God not only created the universe in accordance with the relational love of the Trinity: his love grounds and permeates its order.

4.1.4 Goodness of creation

Augustine's understanding that God created the universe according to the *love* of the Trinity necessarily means that value must be attributed to the whole that is creation as well as to all of its parts. Whatever is, is good. This idea of God's being as love and goodness as underpinning creation is central to Augustine's understanding of creation and human nature as good. God willed the creative word to be in accordance with his goodness. "Whatever things exist, they are good,"[408] Augustine says, and refers it to the Genesis story.

---

402 The understanding of the order of nature is developed further by Oliver O'Donovan, *Resurrection and Moral Order*, in particular 31–38 .
403 Augustine, *City of God*, XI/16.
404 Macqueen, "Contemptus Dei", 232.
405 Augustine, *City of God*, XIX/13.
406 Augustine, *City of God*, XII/5, cf. Macqueen, "Contemptus Dei", 230–237.
407 Augustine, *City of God*, XI/10, cf. Macqueen, "Contemptus Dei", 234.
408 Augustine, *Confessions*, VII/xii/18.

"How are we to understand what is said in every case, that 'God saw that it was good', other than as an approbation of a work made according to the plan which is the wisdom of God? [...] Nothing would have been made had it not been known by Him to be good."[409]

Being and goodness are reciprocal terms: existence can be translated into goodness and vice versa. The Creator and his creation are good. Nevertheless, being absolute goodness, God is "most mightily and incomparably superior to these things"[410] which he created.

God's love and goodness are *in* this world but also *outside* it and *over* it, for God subsists independently of it. According to Augustine's view of God's absolute being, the world is natural, dependent and finite, and is substantially different from God who is supernatural, self-sufficient and infinite. Understanding God through the incarnation and resurrection stories as the one who *loves* the whole of his creation, Augustine sees creation as the realm in which God *materialised* his love. It gives value to its content without ever identifying creation, the natural, with God's love, the supernatural.

Augustine's belief in creation *ex nihilo* and of existence as good entails the rejection of the Manichean doctrine of the present material world as evil in which fragments of divinely originated spirit are trapped – a doctrine to which Augustine himself had adhered for over nine years. According to the Manichees, the passages of Genesis refer to the creation of the material world out of pre-existing matter by the power of evil which resides in the kingdom of darkness. They interpret Genesis 1:2 and the prevailing of darkness as references to the god who rules in the kingdom of darkness, who is the evil god of matter[411] and who struggles against the good god of the spirit. The Manichees believed in "an invasion of the good – the 'Kingdom of Light' – by a hostile force of evil, equal in power, eternal, totally separate – the 'Kingdom of Darkness'"[412] the beginnings of which are accounted for in Genesis.

Although in *The City of God* Augustine argues his doctrine of creation from Genesis, his idea of the goodness of creation is usually ascribed to his Platonism, derived from the account of ontological goodness in Plato's *Timaeus*, where Plato discusses a divine origin of the world and considers the phenomena of nature in relation to it. For Plato, God is good and wished all things to be as good as possible, that is, "to be as like himself as possible". In the *Timaeus*, Plato states "the reason why the frame of this universe of change framed it at all. He was good, and what is good has no particle of envy in it; being therefore without envy he wished all things to be as like himself as possible."[413] Augustine was introduced to Neo-Platonism (as based on the teaching of Plotinus who interpreted Plato) in Milan shortly before his conversion to Christianity.[414]

---

409 Augustine, *City of God*, XI/21.
410 Augustine, *Confessions*, VII/v/7.
411 Weber, *De Genesi contra Manichaeos*, 303–304.
412 Brown, *Augustine*, 47.
413 Plato, *Timaeus*, I/4.
414 Brown, *Augustine*, 88–100.

Regarding Augustine's use of Plato, three points are important to make. First, due to a lack of availability of resources in the world of Greco-Roman antiquity, as Rist points out, "In the late twentieth century we know more about the thought of Plato, Aristotle, Plotinus and the Stoics than he [Augustine] did."[415] What he read may have amounted to a number of books written by other Platonists, only some of them by Plotinus himself.[416] Secondly, there never was one single version of Plato and Plotinus on the philosophical market place of the ancient world. Platonism therefore can mean very different things. Inevitably, Augustine's own approach was subject to his individual concerns such as the exegesis of Scripture in disputes with the Manichees, Donatists or Pelagians. Not sharing the modern scholar's interest in reconstructing the historical philosopher, he used his version of Platonic ideas whenever they seemed to be "the perfect image of what he thought without knowing, or rather, of what he wanted to think and could not."[417] And thirdly, Augustine's aim was first and foremost the understanding of the world from the perspective of Christian revelation. "In particular, his task was to rethink the meanings of time and eternity, nature and history, body and soul, good and evil, in the light of the truth that God is the Creator"[418] who is the Father, Son and Holy Spirit. Neo-Platonism provided him with both a *method* of inquiry and the *vocabulary* for wording his thoughts, whereas the scriptures were the *starting point* of any inquiry as well as its *answers*.

So, Augustine's assertion of the goodness of being is expressed in terms familiar to Plato, yet is not metaphysically akin to it. It is rooted in the testimony of the scriptures. For Augustine, God is, and therefore is good. The Platonic author of the universe is not first and above all *being*, he is not "I am he who is." His goodness comes before his being. He *is*, for he is *good*. According to J.F.Anderson in *Augustine and Being*, Augustine's metaphysics is essentially Christian in that there is no category above *being*: "In a Christian metaphysics, what-is is one, good, true etc., because it is, and not conversely."[419] For Plato, god is *good* and therefore is, whereas for Augustine God primarily *is* and therefore is good. The primacy of being is the essential metaphysical difference between the Christian ontology of Augustine and the philosophical ontology of Plato. In this sense, Augustine's ontology is biblical,[420] so that to ascribe Augustine's, and therefore a large extent of the Western tradition's theorising to the philosophical tradition of Platonism would mean overlooking the driving impulse behind the Augustinian emphasis on the goodness of the material world: understanding the *who is* of the Hebrew Bible, incarnate in the Son of the New Testament.

Having looked at Augustine's analysis of the *who is* and the *what he created*, I now turn to the *whom he created* – the human creature in body and soul, who is the context for the following reflection on disease and health. I start with his view

---

415 Rist, *Augustine*, 1.
416 Ibid., 3.
417 Pegis, "Mind of Augustine", 23/24.
418 Christian, "Creation", 317.
419 Anderson, "Augustine and Being", 5.
420 Ibid., 35.

of the body and its intrinsic goodness, which he explicated above all on the basis
of Christ's incarnation and resurrection.

4.2 THE MATERIAL BODY

Augustine never strove for a glorification of the soul at the cost of the body or
vice versa. Later in his life, when the question of the origin of the soul had become "inflamed and dangerous"[421] in the Pelagian controversy, he defended the
view that both body and soul owed their being to God, the absolute good, and that
therefore both needed to be good.[422] Augustine compares the material body and
the immaterial soul to a couple: he speaks of the "sweet companionship of the
flesh and soul."[423] Human life is always lived in the union of body and soul, of
"the outer man"[424] and the inner man. The monism of an outer-inner man or body-
soul union is central to Augustine's anthropology: due to his firm belief in this
union he "became almost as hostile to 'spiritual' reductionism as he had been
since his conversion to 'material' reductionism."[425]

   This section looks at Augustine's view of the human body, which he approaches from the perspective of its union with the soul. I give examples of Augustine's imagining the union with reference to the incarnation of Christ whose
persona unites divine and human nature, and to his resurrection which re-affirms
the body-soul union. The resurrection is central, too, for Augustine's affirmation
of the goodness of the created body in its state after the Fall.

   Augustine's is a vision and recognition of bodily life that draws its content
from the distinctive understanding of the material world as created and good, and
of its affirmation and future transformation in the resurrection. Augustine developed this vision of the human body as of value and moral significance in the particular context of the gospel of Jesus Christ.

4.2.1 The body in union with the soul

Neo-Platonist idealism tended to identify what it took to be *truly* human with the
immaterial soul, in particular its rational part. The body belonged to the material
world and was considered a liability that might impede the soul's search for happiness and the virtuous life. Individual bodies were seen as vehicles of the soul,
which drew the soul away from the life of the higher and eternal realm to which it
ultimately belonged.[426] The Manichean belief in material creation as related to the
evil creator and ruler of the kingdom of darkness represented the most extreme

421 O'Connell, *Soul in St. Augustine's Later Works*, 246.
422 Teske, "Augustine's Theory of Soul", 120–121.
423 Augustine, *Letters* 140/6/16.
424 Augustine, *Trinity*, XII/1/1.
425 Rist, *Augustine*, 101.
426 Edwards, "Neoplatonism", 588.

form of hostility towards the body in Augustine's time. Originating in the realm of light or the good creation, the human soul was trapped in the human body and was now fighting for its release.[427]

It was in the context of these philosophies – Neo-Platonism and Manicheism – that Augustine set out to explicate biblically the union of body and soul, and the goodness of the human body. He first mentions the body-soul union in 387 when he wrote *The Catholic and the Manichean Way of Life*. Here he states,

> "For although they are two things, soul and body, neither could be called man were the other not present (for the body would not be man if there were no soul, nor would the soul be man were there no body animated by it)."[428]

Twenty years later, in *The Trinity*, he says that the incarnation of Christ shows first, the union of body and soul in humans, second, the precedence of soul over body and, third, the subordination of both to God's word. Christ had shown to the human being

> "What place he would occupy in the things that God has established, seeing that human nature could be so united with God as to become one person from two substances, and, therefore, He is now made up of three: God, the soul, and the flesh."[429]

In this sense, the union of body and soul is hierarchical, as it was for Tatian, Tertullian, and Basil. However, when Augustine says that the body has a mediating function in transmitting messages from the exterior to the interior world of a human being, which the soul deciphers, the union is described in functional terms, with a soul responsible for interior order, and a body responsible for communication with the exterior world.[430]

In the *City of God*, Augustine confirms that humans are composite beings, that is, "not a body alone nor a soul alone; rather [...] composed of both soul and body."[431] This composition is "a miraculous combination"[432] beyond human comprehension, yet also beyond separation. Whoever wanted to separate soul and body would be only testifying to his own madness, Augustine says. Though body and soul are decisively different, they are harmoniously and intrinsically united to form the human being.[433] As John Rist points out,

> "From the time of his conversion, Augustine wished to maintain *both* that it is a man's soul which is created in the image of God, *and* that man himself is some kind of composite of two substances, a soul and a body."[434]

This "mixture of soul and body" forms the human person[435] analogously to the *persona* of Christ which is the union of the divine and human nature.[436]

---

427 Coyle, "Manicheism", 522.
428 Augustine, *Way of Life*, 4/6.
429 Augustine, *Trinity*, XIII/17/22.
430 See Ibid., XI/2.
431 Augustine, *City of God*, XIII/24; X/29; *Trinity*, XI/2/3.
432 Augustine, *City of God*, XXII/24
433 Rist, *Augustine*, 94.
434 Ibid.
435 Ibid.

On account of the union of body and soul, death for Augustine always remained "the most bitter sign of human frailty. For death frustrated the soul's deepest wish which was to live at peace with its beloved, the body."[437] In contrast to the Manichean teaching, Augustine emphasised that death could be never welcomed "as a freeing of the soul from a body."[438] The pains of death arise because the soul is torn away from its natural companion:

> "The death of the body, the separation of the soul from the body, is not good for anyone, as it is experienced by those who are, as we say, dying. This violent sundering of the two elements, which are conjoined and interwoven in a living being, is bound to be a harsh and unnatural experience as long as it lasts."[439]

Even though the soul is torn away in death, it still clings to the body in love. Due to the soul's abiding love, bodies remain personalised bodies, *my* or *your* body. They should never be scorned or cast away after death. A dead body still is the father's body, Augustine stresses in *The City of God* regarding a father's burial:

> "If such things as a father's clothes, and his rings, are dear to their children in proportion to their affection for their parents, then the actual bodies are certainly not to be treated with contempt, since we wear them in a much closer and more intimate way than any clothing."[440]

Ultimately, the doctrine of the resurrection re-affirms the union of body and soul in Augustine's theology.

> "St. Augustine tries to express a single fundamental truth: man is at one and the same time soul *and* body, flesh *and* spirit; and if man is to be truly saved his salvation must embrace his whole being, and therefore the body must also, by glorious resurrection, be taken up into eternity."[441]

In emphasising the transformation which human bodies will undergo in the resurrection, Augustine reminds his readers that (a) it is the *body* that is resurrected and that (b) the resurrected body always remains the very same, personal body. The idea of the survival of human individuality "has become familiar to modern man" yet was "perhaps first realised by St. Augustine,"[442] as Augustinian scholar Henri Marrou remarks. He continues,

> "To say that our individuality continues to exist is also to affirm the perdurance of the entire fabric, woven throughout the whole of our life by the complex of relationships established between our deepest self and God, between ourselves and our human brethren, and finally, between us and the world where we have acted, reacted, struggled, suffered, and created."[443]

---

436 Ibid., 100.
437 Brown, *Body and Society*, 405.
438 Ibid.
439 Augustine, *City of God*, XIII/6.
440 Ibid., I/13.
441 Marrou, *Resurrection and Human Values*, 16.
442 Ibid., 28.
443 Ibid., 29.

4.2.2 Goodness and fallen-ness of the body

Soma, the New Testament's term for body in contrast to *sarx*,[444] describes the body as the material and biological dimension of human life. Humans enter the world as bodies and it is these very same bodies that are buried, that decay and undergo transformation into a different kind of natural matter. How did Augustine view matter? Augustine refers to the body as the outer man and introduces this term in reference to 2 Cor. 4:16. The outer man comprises qualities humans share with all other creatures, not only bodily qualities.

> "It is correctly said, that whatever we have in our soul, in common with the beasts, pertains to the outer man, since by the outer man we mean not the body alone, but also its own peculiar kind of life, whence the structure of the body and all the senses derive their vigour, and by which they are equipped to perceive external things."[445]

Human and other animal creatures share qualities such as sense perception, basic memorial functions or emotive decisions.

> "Even beasts can perceive corporeal things outwardly through the senses of the body, can recall them when they are fixed in the memory, can seek for what is beneficial in them, and flee from what is unpleasant."[446]

These qualities belong to the outer man. They are located in that part of the soul which is shared by humans and other animals: *anima*, the animating principle which marks all creatures as *terra animata*, animated earth.[447] They are *terra* as they are natural; they are *animata* as they are alive, individuated, and physiologically particular.

In contrast to both Neo-Platonist idealism and Manichean radicalism as two ends of a spectrum of hostility towards the body, Augustine interpreted the writings of both the Hebrew Bible and the New Testament as affirming the material body. This is what Peter Brown has in mind when he refers to Augustine as proposing a "markedly different exegesis" of Genesis, that is, of creation and the Fall. As bodies, humans and other animals share material, physical, and sexual characteristics. As bodies, they testify to "the goodness of God, of the providence of the mighty Creator."[448] In humans, such providence can be recognised in the way in which sense organs and body parts are arranged, or in the mobility of tongue and hands, which adapt humans to speaking and writing, the arts and crafts.[449] Augustine refused to read the mythology of the Fall as suggesting that Adam and Eve had fallen from an angelic and spiritual state into a physical state of existence. He did not see humans as essentially spiritual creatures "to whom physical, sexual

---

444 Whilst the term body or *soma* is used more descriptively, the term flesh or *sarx* is also used pejoratively when operating on a moral level ("the flesh lusts against the spirit") yet sometimes also designates man in his totality ("and the Word was made flesh") and then operates on a mainly ontological level. Cf. Schweizer, *'sarx'*, 123–151/*'soma'*, 1054–1091.
445 Augustine, *Trinity*, XII/1/1.
446 Ibid., XIII/2/2.
447 Augustine, *City of God*, XX/20.
448 Ibid., XXII/24.
449 Ibid.

and social needs had once been irrelevant."[450] God created humans as bodily creatures to embrace the material world.

The mature Augustine defended his view of the good body in the Pelagian controversy against the attacks of Julian of Eclanum (418 onwards), who warned his Italian readers that Augustine still believed with his old Manichean teachers in the dualism of body and soul, in an element of evil which permanently existed in human bodies, and in the hostility towards the body (and sexuality) which this entails.[451] Yet Julian was unable to do justice to Augustine's anthropology as he did not have the same mastery of Manichean doctrine, as Peter Brown remarks:

> "Mani's great *Letter of the Foundation* lay to hand on the bookshelves of Hippo, its margins filled with critical notes: thus equipped, it was as easy for Augustine as it is for a modern scholar of Manichean literature to see the difference between his own system and that of Mani, and to shrug off Julian's accusations as a caricature of both."[452]

In affirming the goodness of material life, Augustine rejected Manichean dualism or incorporealism as plainly "foolish": it contradicted the goodness of creation, which includes all created matter. He continues,

> "The Platonists are not, indeed, so foolish as the Manicheans; for they do not detest earthly bodies as the natural substance of evil. On the contrary, they attribute all the elements of which this visible and tangible world is composed, and their properties, to God the Creator."[453]

Both Platonists and Christians are eager to demonstrate, Augustine thought, "that the body is not the source of life, but that life is given to body by God through the medium of the soul."[454] Yet unlike Christians, Platonists "hold that souls are so influenced by earthly limbs and dying members; that they derive from them their unwholesome desires and fears and joys and sorrows".[455] Augustine firmly rejected such a view. At times, Augustine seems to have Manichean or Platonist tendencies. If so, not because bodiliness is of itself negative, but because of humanity's fallen condition, human labouring under God's punishment for Adam's disobedience (*vide infra*). Overall, Augustine's esteem for the body opposes both Neo-Platonist idealism and Manichean dualism.

Augustine's vision and recognition of bodily life draws its content from the distinctive understanding of the material world as created and good, and of its affirmation in the incarnation, and future transformation in the resurrection. Augustine emphasised that the incarnation and resurrection are the foundation of the Christian understanding of the goodness of the human body and of God's claim upon the human body.[456] "The 'flesh' is so far from being despicable that the Word of God willed to assume it."[457] And in the resurrection the goodness of the

---

450 Brown, *Body and Society*, 405.
451 Brown, *Augustine*, 393–394.
452 Ibid., 393.
453 Augustine, *City of God*, XIV/5.
454 Miles, *Plotinus*, 133.
455 Augustine, *City of God*, XIV/5.
456 Cf. I Corinthians 6:12 ff.
457 Marrou, *Resurrection and Human Values*, 13.

human body has been finally affirmed.[458] In its transformed condition the risen body will consist of the same material components as the earthly body: not one hair will perish. "We must not allow ourselves to believe that they will be spirits; we must think of them as bodies having the substance of flesh."[459] The risen body will be reshaped into its most perfect possible form[460] and will be developed to its mature perfection.[461] Every organ and particle it now possesses will be retained. Even the saints will inhabit their very earthly bodies thus paying final tribute to the goodness of the Creator, Augustine believes. After their resurrection, humans will be able to enjoy the beauty of their bodies for its own sake.[462] Bodies will possess the substance of flesh but will be untainted by any carnal corruption and will be completely subdued to the spirit.[463] The resurrection will bring about the disappearance of whatever affliction the body has had to suffer; only that which had positive reality will enter into eternity.

I now turn to the second member of the psychosomatic union – the human soul. I will explore its *relational, dynamic,* and *proleptic* nature, a vision which Augustine developed in the context of the doctrine of the *imago Dei,* the "cornerstone of Augustinian anthropology."[464]

4.3 THE HUMAN SOUL

Reflections on the nature of the entity referred to as "self, spirit, soul, psyche, subjectivity, subject, inner man, person"[465] form a large part of Western philosophy. The terminology of this idea is as inexact as the approaches taken to the question of the entity itself. Often terms are used interchangeably and as indicative of one same reality. For the twentieth century Swiss theologian Karl Barth, the pairs of terms such as "'man as spirit and substantial organism', as 'rational and sensuous', 'inner and outer', 'invisible and 'visible', 'inapprehensible and apprehensible', 'intelligible and empirical' and even as 'heavenly and earthly'",[466] are all indicative of the same reality of *bodily* particularity. Barth himself chooses the pair *body and soul,* for it keeps

> "Us closest to the language of the Bible, and because in their popular simplicity they indicate not only most unpretentiously but also, for all the problems which they involve, most unambiguously, concretely, and comprehensively the questions which are here to be asked and answered."[467]

---

458 Augustine, *City of God,* XIII/23.
459 Ibid.
460 Ibid., XXII/19.
461 Ibid., XXII/14; XXII/15.
462 Ibid., XXII/24.
463 Ibid.
464 Sullivan, *Image of God,* ix.
465 Zaner, "Context and Reflexivity", 154.
466 Barth, *Church Dogmatics,* III/2, 326.
467 Barth, *Church Dogmatics,* III/2, 326.

Augustine identified the specifically human part of the soul with the *imago Dei*. An inquiry into the human soul means inquiring into his understanding of what it means for humans *to be in the image and likeness of God*. Since God is absolute goodness and love, it means inquiring into being in the *image and likeness of his goodness and love*. Such inquiry is, then, the aim of the next two sections.

In view of the study's overall context of health and healing, the aim is not to offer a comprehensive analysis of St Augustine's *imago* doctrine or a complete account of Augustine's view of the human soul, its creation, and functions. Instead, I will look at three particular aspects of Augustine's interpretation of the *imago*, namely, the relational, dynamic, and proleptic aspects, which have implications for his view of health, as well as medical healing and morality. The following inquiry will include looking at Augustine's interpretation of the Fall as the image of God's love as "discoloured" and in need of renewal.

Augustine does not treat the doctrine of the *imago Dei* systematically, but returns to it in various letters, sermons, exegetical and polemical works. He does not achieve a systematic exposition; rather his writings take the form of meditations on the personal-particular and social nature of human life from the perspective of God's love. He does not claim to have penetrated exhaustively what he considers highest mysteries.

Apart from Augustine's own work, I rely upon research undertaken in the past by linguists, historians, philosophers, patristic scholars and theologians, above all J. Heijke's 1960 anthology *St. Augustine's Comments on "Imago Dei" (Exclusive of the De Trinities)*, John E. Sullivan's 1963 *The Image of God – The Doctrine of St. Augustine and its Influence*, R.A.Markus' and G.B.Lander's articles on the image and its reformation (1964/1954), as well as A.-G.Haman's 1987 *L'homme, image de Dieu – essay d'une anthropologie chrétienne dans l'église des cinq premiers siècles*.

4.3.1 Imagining the soul and the image of God

How does Augustine use the term soul? One is confronted here, John Sullivan says, with a fine example of "the fluid Augustinian terminology."[468] Augustine conceives of an incorporeal soul, *anima*, in all living beings, and refers to *all* living entities as *terra animata*.[469] In humans, he distinguishes (1) *anima*, which is both the vegetative part of the soul common to humans, beasts and plants as well as the sentient part common to humans and beasts (that which animates the body); (2) *animus* or *ratio, intellectus, intelligentia, mens humana* or *mens*, which refer to the rational part of the human soul (that which dominates the body). At times, Augustine also calls this part "the eyes of the soul", its "head" or "face".[470] *Animus* and equivalent terms refer not only to human reason but embrace for Au-

---

468 Sullivan, *Image of God*, 64.
469 Augustine, *City of God*, XX/20.
470 Sullivan, *Image of God*, 64 ff.

gustine "*all* of the specifically human and rational activity, and the corresponding faculties."[471] They refer to the "inner man" of Pauline theology,[472] which Augustine understands as "an entity whose activities underlie the being and behaviour of the body in such a way as to make the difference between merely physical activity and the conscious, animated, meaningful, purposive behaviour characteristic of living human beings."[473]

Augustine qualifies the "entity" of the inner man as the site of the *imago Dei* in humans: humans are made in the image of God neither according to the body nor according to any part of the soul but according to the specifically human part of the soul where the knowledge of, and capacity for, God's love resides.[474] Indeed, as God is love and goodness, the image of God in humans is the image of his love. To carry this love "inwardly" is God's inalienable *gift* to the human creature: this is what the story of creation, incarnation and resurrection shows. In being "inward" – inside the specifically human part of the soul, the inner man – God's love is intrinsically present in all humans; through an inwardly turned gaze, humans can recognise this love (God's image) within them. On the basis of this inward presence, the knowledge of God's love is always possible for humans.[475]

Now, how does Augustine understand the specifically human part of the soul on the basis of its being the site of God's image? The inalienable, inward presence of God's love is the foundation of both the personal-particular and social nature of human life. Augustine's thoughts run thus: God is absolute love. As love, he loves every single one of his human creatures as a particular creature. In turn, the creature loves him: Augustine thinks it is a natural desire to love *love*. Humans know whom to love, namely God, as they carry the image of his love inside them. On the basis of this love, they also know to love themselves (for God loves them as particular selves) and their neighbours (whom God loves as particular selves). One loves in one self and in the other the presence of God's love. Where we love our brothers, we love the same love so that the love of self and neighbour is nothing but the love of love, of God's love (*amor amoris*).[476] God's love is *qualified* love: it is qualified through the life of Christ. This is, then, the root of Augustine's relational vision of the soul.

How does Augustine's view of the soul and the *imago Dei* compare with other interpretations? The doctrine of the *imago Dei* is derived from the book of Genesis. Here, man and woman are affirmed to be in the image (*selem*) of God, and in his likeness (*d'mut*). Scriptural exegesis of this passage is concerned mainly with the meaning of the terms image and likeness in Hebrew, the origins of these terms, and their possible meaning in the passage and in the wider context of Genesis.

St Paul uses the term image (*eikon*) in reference to Christ: Christ being the image of God. He also uses it to describe the process of a person's movement in

---

471 Sullivan, *Image of God*, 64 ff.
472 Ibid., 45–49.
473 Matthews, "Inner Man", 187.
474 Augustine, *Literal Interpretation of Genesis*, 3.20.30; *Trinity*, XII/7/12.
475 Augustine, *Trinity*, VIII/11.
476 Ibid., VIII/10.

life towards eschatological fullness as one of becoming more conformed to the image of the Son;[477] in this sense the image of God is indicative of the glory that awaits humans in the future life.

In his principal work *Adversus Haereses*, Irenaeus of Lyon (140–202) was perhaps the first theologian to offer a detailed interpretation of Genesis 1:26, which also became the anchor of his theology as a whole. A complete Latin translation of his work was available as early as 421, when Augustine may well have read it, too.[478] An image for Irenaeus was a bodily reality,[479] which is visibly able to reveal and represent its exemplar or archetype: "Irenaeus found the image in the human body, modelled after the flesh of Christ, who was to restore the likeness lost by sin."[480] Image, he said, points to the visible human nature, the *homo imperfectus*, of which the future Christ was the model, whereas likeness indicates the *homo perfectus* who is modelled by the Spirit.[481] Likeness was lost in the event of the Fall and needed to be regained. The human image of God in contrast is inalienable. Likeness presupposes being-in-the image and adds, when realised, something to the image.[482] Likeness is dynamic, whereas image is static.[483] Likeness develops and grows under the influence of the Holy Spirit.

Following Irenaeus' reading of Genesis 1:26, some of Augustine's contemporaries from both the East and West, such as Cyril of Alexandria and Ambrose, reserved the term image for natural human endowments (modelled after Christ), and likeness for supernatural gifts (modelled by the Spirit).[484] Scholastic theologians, too, distinguished between image as a term of correspondence describing the ontological nature of human life and likeness as being realised in one's relationship to God.[485]

Augustine repudiates the distinction found in the Greek tradition where likeness adds something new to the idea of being in the image and where it is thought of as goal of human development. Image and likeness, though distinguishable philosophically,[486] are synonyms in the account of Genesis. Image and likeness were both there from the beginning as identifying that which is specifically human in the soul: the relationship of love between God, the self, and the other. What changed with the Fall was the *degree of likeness* between the image and the original: the Fall caused a disturbance in the relation between God (the original) and the specifically human part of the soul (the image). After the Fall,

---

477 Rom 8:29/2 Cor 3:18.
478 Clark, "Irenaeus", 457.
479 Hamman, *Image de Dieu*, 67.
480 Clark, "Irenaeus", 457.
481 Irenaeus, *Against Heresies*, V/6/1.
482 This is what the Greek term for 'likeness' (*homoousis*) suggests according to Markus, "Imago and Similitudo", 126.
483 Cf. Markus, "Imago and Similitudo", 126/141.
484 Sullivan, *Image of God*, 12.
485 Joest, *Dogmatik II*, 354.
486 Hamman, *Image de Dieu*, 256.

the image of God in humans, the vision of his love in the human soul, is "impaired and disfigured"[487] and needs to be reformed.

We indeed recognise in ourselves the image of God: that is, of the supreme Trinity. This image is not equal to God. Indeed it is very far removed from Him; for it is neither co-eternal with Him, nor, to express the whole matter briefly is it of the same substance as God. It is, however, nearer to God in nature than any-thing else made by Him, *even though it still requires reforming and perfecting in order to be a still closer likeness.*[488]

Due to the Fall, humans are unable to see God's love clearly. God's love has not changed, as He is immutable; its presence within humans has become less clearly visible. As a consequence, humans fail to understand the personal and social dimension of life, and its implications for human action. The one purpose of Christ's coming (and dying) is to reveal God's love once more, and hence, to allow for the restoration of the image of love in humans. For Augustine, Christ's coming allows humans to love *love* again, and on this basis, to recognise what it means to live a good and fulfilled life as persons in social relationships.

4.3.2 The soul and the reformation of the imago

Augustine understands the soul to be in need of *renewal*.[489] It needs to be refor-med, not re-created. Here, Augustine's view of degrees of likeness is important: a human being's likeness to God's goodness has not been lost. It has not been *wiped out,* as being itself has not been wiped out. Augustine uses the metaphor "discol-oured".[490] The specifically human part of the soul (that which is in the image of God's love and which is capable of relationship with God) has been discoloured so that it does not show the colour of God's love anymore. As a consequence, they cannot relate to God. And without foregoing clarification of the image they cannot act morally, since moral action is oriented to God's love. Hence, the re-newal of the image of God is foundational for morality. It is a process initiated gratuitously by God in Christ, as an initiative that works on an existing being.[491]

Against this background, the specifically human part of the soul is not a static or fixed entity but describes an entity 'in progress', on its way. The soul is in the process of renewing its relationship with God, in movement towards his love, and towards closer likeness to his goodness. In this process, it moves towards its own goodness and fullness.

Inquiring into the dynamic and prolepsis aspect of the soul ('its specifically human part'), two aspects need to be more closely looked at: (1) the Fall as moral event due to which the image of God requires renewal and (2) the role of Christ and the Holy Spirit in the process of the restoration of the image of God in hu-

---

487 Augustine, *Trinity*, XIV/8/11.
488 Augustine, *City of God*, XI/26 (my italics).
489 Augustine, *Trinity*, XII/7/10.
490 Augustine, *Ex 3 of Ps* XXXII/16.
491 Ibid.

mans. Both aspects are central to Augustine's anthropology and are foundational for his view of health and healing.

(1) Augustine understands the Genesis myth as historical. It accounts for humanity's origin in the first human couple, Adam and Eve – another root of humanity's social nature.[492] In the pre-Fallen state, Adam was both mortal and immortal: mortal, for he could die, immortal for he could also not die – depending on his obedience to the Creator.[493] The initial freedom that is contained in the *posse non peccary* was thwarted by Adam and Eve's disobedience. In violating God's law not to eat fruits of the tree of knowledge Adam and Eve set themselves outside the order instituted by the Creator. They did not understand their distinct place within the order of creation; ignoring God's law, they were ignorant of the fact that they had been made so that it was to their advantage to be subject to God, and that it was harmful to act according to their own will.[494] Instead of a *conversion ad Deum*, Genesis accounts for the human aversion of God and their *conversion ad creatures*.

At the root of Adam and Eve's desire for independence was their soul's pride,[495] a desire of elevation of the self.[496] A proud soul only knows a perverted kind of love: not the love of God that belongs to the order of nature, and of which humans carry the image, but the love of the self, which opposes the order of nature and the love of God. The desire to elevate one's self is the beginning of all sin: this psychology is at the heart of what Augustine wants to get at in his exegesis of Genesis. It also exposes what he considers to be the true nature of Manichaean theodicy: the elevation of self above God.

Human pride originates from a defect in the human will, which in turn has its roots in the creation *ex nihilo*. "This I know: that the nature of God cannot ever, anywhere or in any way, be defective, whereas natures made out of nothing can be."[497] A substance that has been created out of nothing, Augustine says, has an inherent tendency towards the non-existence out of which it was brought into the goodness of existence. Against the Manichees, evil is not ascribed to the influence of an enemy of the divine Creator trying to rule over the human creature. The creature turns against the Creator from its own will. "It is the defection of the will itself which is evil [...]. It is a turning away from that which has supreme being and towards that which has less."[498] Having its cause in the soul's disobedience, the Fall is first of all an internal and moral event, which has external and physical effects such as pain, illness and death, and a distortion of the (also sexual) appetites. These effects are God's punishment for the Fall.[499] All human generations

---

492 See for instance Augustine, *City of God*, XII/22 or XII/28.
493 Augustine, *Literal Interpretation of Genesis*, 6.24.36.
494 Augustine, *City of God*, XIV/12.
495 Augustine, *Trinity*, XII/9/14.
496 Augustine, *City of God*, XIV/13.
497 Ibid., XII/8.
498 Augustine, *City of God,* XII/8.
499 Gen. 3.

inherited this condition: they are in a state of original sin, and suffer from its effects.[500]

(2) For Augustine, the history of humanity takes place in the grip of sin and the advent of grace: in Christ, the incarnation of the Word of God, humans are able to re-discover the image of God disfigured in Adam. The *imago Dei* is renewed in particular through God's grace working in the sacraments of baptism. In Augustine's words,

> "This renewal, of course, is not brought about in the one moment of the conversion itself, as in Baptism that renewal is brought about in one moment by the remission of sins, for there does not remain even one sin, however small it may be, that is not forgiven. But just as it is one thing to be free from fevers, and another thing to recover from the weakness which has resulted from the fevers; and, similarly, just as it is one thing to remove a spear that has been driven into the body, and another thing to heal the wound that has been made by it through the treatment that follows, so the first step in a cure is to remove the cause of the disease, which is done through the remission of all sins; the second is to heal the disease itself, which is done gradually by making progress in the renewal of this image."[501]

In the context of the Pelagian controversy and their belief in human ability to reform oneself and the world independently of grace, Augustine expressed a view that holds the renewal of the image to be worked in two stages: in the moment of baptism, individual sins and inherited sin are forgiven. Then, in her daily life and work, a person progresses spiritually, she grows in resemblance to God's love, and in this moves towards her own full human-ness. Against the Pelagians, Augustine was extremely careful to emphasise that *grace* does not minimise human activity. On the contrary: it wakes human senses, it transforms the human soul in faith, hope and charity, and it fills the human being with a longing desire for accomplishment, rest and peace.[502]

Augustine drew a clear distinction between *baptismal* and *post-baptismal* regeneration, showing that the initial renewal conferred at baptism is instantaneous yet that moral efforts and active participation in God's love needed to follow. This distinction enabled Augustine to establish a

> "Balance between God's grace and man's will, between the sacraments and morality, which was to become the theological foundation of all Christian reform movements in the west for a thousand years. He did so by stressing the role of the divine reformer Christ over that of man the reformer, and on the other hand by insisting on the necessity of continuous reform in human life."[503]

The gradual renewal of the image means that humans grow in resemblance to God in the restored knowledge of his love, and with God's gracious love being the effective principle in this process.[504]

---

500 Augustine, *City of God*, XIII/3.
501 Augustine, *Trinity*, XIV/17/23.
502 Hamman, *Image de Dieu*, 272.
503 Ladner, "Conception of Reformation", 871.
504 Augustine, *Trinity*, XIV/17/23.

Finally, the renewal of the human soul is *not* simply to a pristine state, Augustine said, but to something greater. The final perfection of the divine image in humans occurs in the state of beatitude and consists in the fullness of the vision of God.

> "Man's reform to the better was achieved by Christ's assuming in the Incarnation the form of a servant, by redeeming us through His death from servitude to sin and death, and by thus bestowing on us something which Adam had *not* had; namely, immortality."[505]

This final renewal happens in the resurrection, which "is therefore a fuller, a better state, incomparably superior to anything we have known or experienced during our earthly life."[506] In a sense, the *imago Dei* in the specifically human part of the soul is prolepsis: it foreshadows and anticipates the fullness of life to be experienced in the eschatological future.

4.3.3 Concluding remarks

According to Augustine, the *imago Dei* indicates the distinct *relationship* of love between the Creator and the human creature. It indicates it as inalienable and intrinsic to the human soul, and to everything that is particular or personal about the human creature. In their souls, God addresses humans; they are called into relationship with him. In God's address of the soul, the human being is recognised as a *particular* human being. God's love directs this particular being to his or her fellow humans who are also loved by God, so that in the neighbour, one loves God's love. This address of the self and call into relationship with the other is possible because the image of God in the human soul has not been wiped out. Due to the Fall human particularity cannot be fully recognised, and social life cannot be fully realised. Through grace both human personhood and sociability will be reformed, ultimately (in the eschaton) to the fullest goodness in which humans may exist.

In the context of his mature reading of the *imago Dei*, the soul for Augustine clearly embraces ontological qualities which constitute the difference between humans and beasts, such as reason, self-awareness, free will, and the capacity for meaningful decision-making. Yet above all, the soul of a human being is the site of the relational process between the creature and the Creator, and between the creature and her fellow-creatures.

The *imago Dei* doctrine indicates the relationship of love between the Creator and the human creature as foundation for understanding particularity or personal identity. Personal identity includes sociability, and is discerned in fraternal interaction: through the love of God, a particular human being is directed to his or her fellow humans. The *imago* doctrine indicates the Creator-creature relationship as inalienable and intrinsic to the human soul, hence, to everything that is particular or personal about the human creature.

---

505 Ladner, "Conception of Reformation", 368.
506 Marrou, *Resurrection and Human Value*, 22.

The personhood one discerns fraternally according to Augustine is indeed *real*, yet it is *not yet* realised in its *fullest sense*. This distinction of *real* and *not fully realised yet* includes all human life be it the life of the embryo, the newborn, the girl or boy, the man or woman: we are all persons, yet not fully realised persons yet. We all are to be valued and protected in a faith expectant of a future, irrespective of measurable and apparent qualities, precisely because personhood will only be realised *and* understood fully in the completion of life in the eschatological future.

The understanding of personhood (as the ways in which the human embryo, the child, the adult are *personal*) requires a mode of deliberation radically different to the world of empirical investigation and scientific facts.[507] The Augustinian mode of deliberation is an inward turn to God's love revealed in Christ, a turn away from outward sense perception and observation of physical appearances.[508] In this sense, Oliver O'Donovan elucidates the idea of personhood not by reference to the objectivity of the laboratory but with the New Testament story of the Good Samaritan.[509] It shows that personhood is a hypothesis which is proved through neighbourly interaction in the first place. Scientific observation drawing on physical appearance says that developmental individuality occurs at around day fourteen; theological observations "do not of themselves yield any very precise view of the beginnings of individual identity."[510] Yet personal identity is not a natural category and cannot be described according to empirical observations, general appearances and measurable performance. It does not belong to the world of observation and natural facts. Personal identity cannot be recognised from the distance of an experiment or in the planned observation of a behavioural test.[511] With Augustine, it can be properly called *mysterious*. Beneath this, it may be called (as it is by O'Donovan) a hypothesis proved through interaction. But interaction is not posterior; it is not based upon the results of scientific testing: one does not need appearance or tests to understand whether the other demands respect. Interaction and inter-subjective relationality is a given in as much as the human soul in its union with the body is a given.

Against the background of this study's overall concern with a framework of health and medical healing grounded in an integrative vision of human life, it is necessary to rest a while with Augustine and to reflect with him, on the basis of the anthropology he developed, on the relationship of diseases of the body and health of the soul, medical healing and God's salvation. I will start by turning to Augustine's interpretation of physical illness as God's punishment for human sin as can be found in *The Confessions, Exposition of the Psalms,* and *The City of God.* I critically analyse this connection in dialogue with John Burnaby's 1938 *Amor Dei* and Albert Camus' 1948 *The Plague.*

---

507 O'Donovan, *Begotten or Made*, 57.
508 Augustine, *Trinity*, XI/1/1.
509 O'Donovan, *Begotten or Made*, 57.
510 Ibid., 56.
511 Ibid., 59.

In the encounter of doctor Rieux and Father Paneloux, the Augustinian scholar, Camus' *Plague* plays out elements of Augustinian theology in a medical context. At times, *The Plague* illustrates Augustine's interpretation; at other times it questions his reading from the perspective of events as they take place in the imaginary city of Oran, aptly situated in North Africa, Augustine's home province. For Albert Camus the city of Oran represents the human condition as such.[512] He shares this assumption with Augustine's use of the city of Rome.

> "It is clear from their respective works that both Augustine and Camus intended to convey universal moral significance rather than particularised description of one or the other geographical city. For both men the city is a symbol of the human race as a moral entity seeking its ends according to the diversity of character of its several members."[513]

Both cities enclose the full range of humanity, from those who exploit suffering to those who put their lives to the service of the suffering of others.

4.4 PHYSICAL DISEASE AND HUMAN SINFULNESS

Augustine knew how it felt to suffer pain, to be ill, to be physically exhausted and worn out. Already as a boy he had come close to death. He recalls in *The Confessions*: "One day, when I was still a small boy, pressure on the chest suddenly made me hot with fever and almost at death's door."[514] As a young man shortly after his arrival in Rome he fell ill from serious fever and once more was "on the way to the underworld."[515] And at what was perhaps the most crucial point in his life, in Milan, before his baptism, his "lungs had begun to weaken. Breathing became difficult. Pains on the chest were symptoms of the lesion, and deprived me of the power to speak clearly for any length of time."[516] Augustine was forced to resign from his teaching post and had to give up hopes of resuming his career as a rhetorician at the imperial court. Even though his lung condition improved after his summer holidays in Cassiacium, other illnesses continued to plague him until the end of his life. As an old man he wrote in a letter to his brother Profuturus,

> "In spirit, as far as it pleases the Lord, and as He deigns to give me strength, I am well, but in body, I am in bed, for I can neither walk nor stand nor sit because of the pain and swelling of haemorrhoids and chafing."[517]

Augustine had also experienced the "bitterness of life"[518] present in the death of others. During his years as a Manichee in Carthage life became burdensome after a close friend died; all that he had shared with him was transformed into a cruel

---

512 Lavère, "Camus and Augustine", 87.
513 Ibid.
514 Augustine, *Confessions*, I/xi/17.
515 Ibid., V/ix/16.
516 Ibid., IX/ii/4.
517 Augustine, *To Profuturus*.
518 Augustine, *Confessions*, IV/v/10.

torment.[519] After the death of his mother in particular "an overwhelming grief welled into my heart and was about to flow forth in floods of tears."[520] He suffered "sharp pains of inward grief"[521] and turned to God to heal his pain,[522] even though he knew that neither had she suffered extinction nor that her new state was miserable.

In Augustine's thought bodily disease, mortality and the doctrine of original sin are closely linked. Disease and death became a part of human life only after the event in the Garden. They are inflicted upon humans as punishment for their sins, both for the inherited state of original sin as well as for sin acquired through voluntary acts of disobedience to God. Not unlike Tertullian, Augustine thought that such punishment would improve and purify, and strengthen humans' faith.

As Camus' *Plague* illustrates, this proposition is difficult to defend where confronted with the physical suffering and dying of children. It misses out, as Burnaby points out, that a *Christian* view of physical disease and suffering focuses on God's self-revelation as the one who suffers with us, overcomes suffering and transforms death into joy and fullness of life.

4.4.1 Disease as divine punishment

The citizens of Oran experience the "bitterness of life" or "*malheur*"[523] on a grand scale. In the face of monumental suffering, the plague, Father Paneloux, the Augustinian scholar and city priest, has as his main concern how the existence of suffering can be reconciled with God's goodness. In the early days of the plague he delivers a sermon to a huge congregation, of which the opening line reads, "Mes frères, vous êtes dans le malheur, mes frères, vous l'avez merité"[524] – "Calamity has come on you, my brethren, and, my brethren, you deserved it."[525] Paneloux continues,

> "If today the plague is in your midst, that is, because the hour has struck for taking thought. The just man need have no fear, but the evil-doer has good cause to tremble. For plague is the flail of God and the world His threshing-floor, and implacably he will thresh out His harvest until the wheat is separated from the chaff. There will be more chaff then wheat, few chosen of the many called. [...] For a long while God gazed down on this town with eyes of compassion; but He grew weary of waiting, His eternal hope was too long deferred, and now He has turned His face away from us. And so, God's light withdrawn, we walk in darkness, in the thick darkness of this plague."[526]

---

519 Augustine, *Confessions*, IV/iv/9.
520 Ibid., IX/xii/29.
521 Ibid., IX/xi/30.
522 Ibid., IX/xii/32.
523 Camus, *La Peste*, 91. The term 'malheur' is rendered 'calamity' in the English translation. 'Misfortune' would be a perhaps more literal translation.
524 Ibid.
525 Camus, *The Plague*, 80.
526 Ibid., 80-81.

In this sermon Father Paneloux most explicitly recalls Augustine in considering the plague as "the flail of God". Augustine came to understand evil (and this includes bodily evil such as disease and death) as divine retribution, as a just punishment for humanity's chosen disobedience to the command of love. For Augustine, humans are of their "own will corrupted and justly condemned".[527]

Death was not a part of human life from the moment of its creation, but only after the event in the Garden. Human mortality is inflicted upon humans as punishment for their sin.

> "The death of the body was not inflicted upon us by law of our nature, since God did not create any death for man in his nature, but it was imposed as a just punishment for sin. For it was when God was taking vengeance on sin that he said to the man, in whom we all existed at that time, 'You are earth, and into earth you will go.'"[528]

Death (and with death, disease and physical suffering) is a penalty, a divine sentence, a just condemnation, an imposed matter of punishment for sin – these are the words Augustine most frequently uses to qualify mortality.[529] As Burnaby remarks on the subject, "Augustine offers his doctrine of original sin as the only tenable explanation of the facts of human suffering. Men's misery proves their guilt."[530]

Augustine's explanation of disease has three main components: (1) God's punishment is *just*. It is just, since the first sinful act was not necessary but voluntary.[531] And how could something that comes from God, who is absolute goodness and justice, be other than good and just? God's anger must be just, for God's being is absolute and unquestionable justice. To hold the opposite is to commit the guilt of accusing God and making excuses for oneself, something for which Augustine continually and passionately rebuked the Manicheans. To doubt God's justice for Augustine meant the refusal to face the moral consequences of sin or to apply lax human standards of justice to God, who transcends all human capacities of understanding. If the first human couple had not sinned, humans would have been rewarded with "angelic immortality and a blessed eternity."[532]

(2) The punishment is not only just but also *inherited*. It is handed down from Adam and Eve to all future generations, to the whole of humanity. As Augustine says in *The City of God,*

> "We must, then, confess that the first human beings were so constituted that, had they not sinned, they would not have experienced any kind of death; but that, having become the first sinners, they were then punished by death in such a way that whatsoever sprang from their stock should also be subject to the same penalty."[533]

(3) Physical disease is not an inherited punishment alone: it is acquired and *earned* where one commits direct, intentional acts of disobedience to God. Such

527 Augustine, *City of God*, XIII/14.
528 Ibid., XIII/15.
529 See for instance Augustine, ibid., XIII.
530 Burnaby, *Amor Dei*, 203.
531 Augustine, *City of God*, XII/9.
532 Ibid., XIII/1.
533 Ibid., XIII/3.

acts of disobedience (or acts of individual sin) flow from the inherited, indirect condition of sinfulness, which left the *imago Dei* discoloured. Here we find Augustine's distinction between anterior bondage and adult concupiscence.

Augustine taught that, first, after the Fall the human will is bound to evil prior to any adult concupiscence. Anterior bondage means that *a priori* humans *are* guilty. Secondly, due to this bondage the human will turns against God in concrete actions. Adult concupiscence describes that in acting humans *become* guilty.[534] Now, physical disease results from both kinds of sinfulness – inherited, and acquired.

Generally speaking, *sin* for Augustine refers to the event of the Fall, and to the subsequent acts of disobedience that place humans outside the order of God's love. Morally good actions have God's love both as their origin and end. Where humans violate the law of love, they set themselves outside the order of things instituted by the Creator. Where they ignore God's law of love, humans do not understand their distinct place within the order of creation.

Yet how could the first human couple, parents of the whole of humanity, fall away from God's love as its source of goodness? As has been shown in the context of the *imago* interpretation, Augustine sought to explain the Fall with reference to the free will with which humans were created, and with reference to an imperfection in that will due to its being created out of nothing. This imperfection or defectiveness means that the human will, though made by the good Creator, is able to negate its own freedom in God and turn to evil. For Augustine createdness implies imperfection, though not iniquity. A substance that has been created out of nothing, Augustine says (and here he draws upon a Neoplatonist understanding of substance), has an inherent tendency towards the non-existence out of which it was brought into the goodness of existence. That tendency towards the non-existence is at the root of all evil action.

It has been suggested that this notion of an intrinsic, and hence inevitable, tendency towards nothingness is problematic. For instance Robert Brown points out in his 1978 article, the "contention that free creatures made 'out of nothing' inevitably fall makes the Fall seem ontologically necessary (unfree) and thereby lays the ultimate responsibility for it on the Creator."[535] How can the will be considered free when it intrinsically tends to evil? Such a contention questions both the Creator's full goodness and the freedom of the human will.

Yet the notion of tendency towards nothingness prevented, and was designed to prevent, ascribing evil to the influence of a real and personal enemy of the Creator, which would have questioned God's omnipotence. Augustine's argument develops in the context of an attack on the Manichean construction of a kingdom of darkness that opposes God's kingdom of light. This Manichean theodicy Augustine exposed as achieving nothing but the preservation of the purity of their own particular Manichaean souls and rational judgments over against God's om-

---

534 Cf. Rigby, "Original Sin", 72.
535 Brown, "First Evil Will", 315 (my italics).

nipotence, opposing their justice to God's justice, their reason to his reason, and their love to his love.

In emphasising that it is of her own free will, deficient due to her being created *ex nihilo*, that the creature turned herself against the Creator, Augustine redresses this Manichaean compromise of God's power for the sake of the soul's purity. The Fall is attributed to an intrinsic human lack – not God's lack.

As such, having its cause in the human will's defect, the Fall is for Augustine first of all an internal and moral event in a moral story; only secondarily does it have external and physical effects such as disease and death. On this basis, Augustine was able to avoid – this time in the context of the Pelagian controversy – a view of the Fall as an entirely ontological event, a view which he had been accused of holding by Julian of Eclanum. As has been discussed earlier, Augustine emphasised that after the Fall both body and soul remained good. As has been concluded earlier, this is what Augustine inferred from the doctrine of the resurrection. The Fall is a moral event with *ontological implications*.

Now, these implications are God's collective punishment for Adam's sin, Augustine said – a view which his adversary Julian saw as a gross caricature of the loving God of Christ's revelation.[536] The conflict with Julian of Eclanum (which Augustine did not live to solve)[537] evolved around the question of God's justice and love in the face of human suffering. Julian's basic premise was that a just God would never count the sin of someone else against children born without sin. Sin for Julian is the action of an independent, adult, rational being.[538]

4.4.2 Physical suffering and redemption

In the city of Oran a little boy's illness and subsequent death raise the question of disease understood as either punishment or innocent suffering in a most acute way. Both doctor Rieux and Tarrou, the reporter of events, have already seen children die,

> "But they had never yet watched a child's agony minute by minute [...]. Needless to say, the pain inflicted on these innocent victims had always seemed to them to be what in fact it was: an abominable thing. But hitherto they had felt its abomination in, so to speak, an abstract way; they had never had to witness over so long a period the death-throes of *an innocent child*."[539]

Having been present at the little boy's death bed and having seen his agony, it is clear for Rieux and Tarrou that children are *innocent victims of illness*. Rieux shouts both in anger and despair at Father Paneloux, "That child, anyhow, was innocent – and you know it as well as I do!"[540] A conversation develops between the doctor and the priest, in which Rieux affirms that for him children are inno-

---

536 Brown, *Augustine*, 391–392.
537 Bonner, "Contra Julianum", 481.
538 Lamberigts, "Julian of Eclanum", 479.
539 Camus, *The Plague*, 174–175 (my italics).
540 Ibid., 177.

cently put to torture in disease and death. This brute fact calls into question the existence of a loving God.

> "Rieux turned towards Paneloux. [...] And there are times when the only feeling I have is one of mad revolt.' 'I understand,' Paneloux said in a low voice. 'That sort of thing is revolting because it passes our human understanding. But perhaps we should love what we cannot understand.' Rieux straightened up slowly. He gazed at Paneloux, summoning to his gaze all the strength and fervour he could muster against his weariness. Then he shook his head. 'No, Father. I've a very different idea of love. And until my dying day I shall refuse to love a scheme of things in which children are put to torture.'"[541]

In the face of the suffering of infants and, perhaps even more acutely, newly born babies, it is brutal to draw a connection between illness and individual acts of disobedience, Rieux implies. Infants and babies do not possess a will which is capable of making its own choices, which would make them morally culpable for their own acts. How can children deserve punishment if they cannot freely reject God's love and choose disobedience to God? This was Julian of Eclanum's question in Augustine's life time. Both Rieux and Julian touch upon classical questions of theodicy: if God is all-powerful and good, how can there be evil in the world? How can bad things happen to innocent people and how can one consider God to be love in the face of suffering? One must compromise God's power (evil exists, so he is not powerful enough to overrule it) and love (evil exists so he is not loving enough to allow for his love as only power), Rieux says.

To this kind of argument, Augustine replied with the distinction between anterior bondage and adult concupiscence. *Original sin* denotes inherited immorality, human guilt from birth. Even where inherited guilt is removed (as is the case in baptism) its effects such as death and disease remain so that from birth onwards, a baby lives under the impending punishment of suffering and death. However, for Augustine the baby is *not* burdened by any of its own wilfully committed acts of sin, so that it awaits "the mildest condemnation" in the afterlife.[542] For Julian of Eclanum, as for doctor Rieux, a God who judges in this way is "the persecutor of new-born children."[543] For Julian such a view of the nature of God is not compatible with the Christian revelation of the good God, who created the universe as good, who loves humanity, and has given his Son for human salvation.[544] For Julian,

> "The punishment of others for the sin of their father, the condemnation of helpless babies, the passing of sentence on men who had been unable to act otherwise; the whole Christian revelation was a measured and authoritative declaration against such *iniquities*, such corrupt dealing."[545]

Yet to Augustine, Julian's idea of God's nature as justice and love was a rationalistic *human* idea of justice[546] which failed to penetrate divine justice. "Whoever

---

541 Camus, *The Plague*, 178.
542 Bonner, "Contra Julianum", 480.
543 Brown, *Augustine*, 391.
544 Ibid.
545 Ibid., 392.
546 Ibid., 393.

thinks such punishment either excessive or unjust shows his inability to measure the great iniquity of sinning where sin might so easily have been avoided."[547] Human misery proves human sin *not* God's injustice. God's justice is as inscrutable to the human mind as any other aspect of his nature. "Julian might use his reason to define a newborn baby as innocent. The eyes of God, in the Scriptures, saw deeper."[548] God for Augustine is absolute goodness, omnipotence, and justice – and "as he is absolutely just, the appalling sufferings of the human race could only be permitted because he was angry."[549]

Against Augustine's interpretation of physical suffering a Christian approach to suffering needs to have at its centre God's love of humanity. This is Father Paneloux's position and the basis of John Burnaby's critique of Augustine's theory of punishment. Before turning to John Burnaby in more detail, I will engage with Father Paneloux in the follow-up to the little boy's death.

For Father Paneloux, suffering is incomprehensible. Faith confronts humans where reason recoils. It touches upon, and develops from, the limit of what can be thought. Children's deaths will always reach beyond the capacity of human understanding. Facing a child's agony, humans face the ultimate choice of faith. Where the boundaries of human reason are reached, they either move beyond these boundaries into the realm where faith is the only source of knowledge, or they hold on to human reason as only source of knowledge. Either they believe everything that has been revealed about God and his love (despite their rational interpretation of events), or they deny everything that lies beyond reason.[550] God's redemptive love lies beyond reason – indeed it confronts it.[551]

After the little boy's death, for Father Paneloux (and against Augustine) the appropriate answer to the question of suffering can only be an *irrational* affirmation of God's love in faith: "Perhaps we should love what we cannot understand."[552] He explains,

> "The love of God is a hard love. It demands total self-surrender, disdain of our human personality. And yet it alone can reconcile us to suffering and the deaths of children, it alone can justify them, since we cannot understand them, and we can only make God's will ours. That is the hard lesson I would share with you to-day. That is the faith, cruel in men's eyes, and crucial in God's, which we must ever strive to compass."[553]

Father Paneloux's position here resembles that of Sören Kierkegaard in *Fear and Trembling*. Kierkegaard characterises faith in God's love by prior resignation.[554] For him, faith enters the scene when humans have renounced rationality. In faith, it is possible to accept God's love as the ultimate end of human life in the face of suffering and death. Similarly, Father Paneloux concludes that suffering cannot be

547 Augustine, *City of God*, XIV/15.
548 Brown, *Augustine*, 393.
549 Ibid., 395.
550 Camus, *The Plague*, 183.
551 Ibid.
552 Ibid., 178.
553 Ibid., 186.
554 Kierkegaard, *Fear and Trembling*, 66/75.

made sense of through rational enquiry and reflection alone. Questions of the causality of evil (which include intricacies such as the defect of the free will), theories of punishment and ultimately the question of theodicy cannot be humans'
primary interest.

Indeed, for a Christian, questions of theodicy and theories of punishment
should not be of any interest in the face of suffering and disease: what matters is
suffering's end and aim. This is, according to John Burnaby, the lesson one has to
learn from a *Christian* reading of the book of Job. For according to a Christian
reading Christ's suffering is the final answer to Job's questioning. In Job, Burnaby
says, "We see a mind of exceptional power and originality rejecting the premiss
that all suffering is the punishment of sin."[555]

A Christian's primary interest needs to be God's love and redemption, John
Burnaby emphasises in *Amor Dei*, a collection of lectures on Augustine first published in 1938. Here, he objects to Augustine's interpretation of suffering which
differs but little from that of Job's comforters. Augustine "failed [...] to reach
anything like a Christian solution of the problem of suffering."[556]

Burnaby's main point in his critique of Augustine's view of suffering and sin
is that "any 'explanation' of suffering must lie not in its beginning but in its
end."[557] Here, Burnaby does *not* refer to the idea in Augustine that the evil of suffering can be used for the patient's good, for instance, for righteousness' sake;[558]
or that the death of body had to remain after baptism for its strengthening impact
on faith;[559] or that "what had been imposed as the penalty for sin had been turned
to such good use that it brought to birth a richer harvest of righteousness."[560]

What Burnaby has in mind when talking about suffering's end is God's abundant love through which all human misery was, is, and will be surpassed. It is,
first and last of all, joy and happiness which God wants for the creature he loves.
It is "the love which brings happiness in refusing the pursuit of pleasure" and
which transfigures pain "without denying its painfulness or stifling the movement
of compassion."[561] God's love, Burnaby says, has been revealed to humans in
Christ's passion and resurrection; through his passion and resurrection the evil has
been wrung out of human suffering.[562] God has revealed himself not only as the
one who is at our side when we suffer, but above all, as the one through whom our
pain is overcome transformed into joy and happiness. This is what needs to be at
the centre of a *Christian* view of suffering according to Burnaby.

Augustine drew his idea of physical punishment from the ordinary assumptions of legal justice in the Roman Empire. Burnaby explains that a social of-
fender must be shown, it was assumed by Roman criminal law,

555 Burnaby, *Amor Dei*, 201.
556 Ibid., 205.
557 Ibid.
558 Augustine, *Patience*, 8/x.
559 Augustine, *City of God*, XIII/4.
560 Ibid., XIII/7.
561 Burnaby, *Amor Dei*, 205.
562 Ibid.

"That wrong-doing does not pay, and the only way of ensuring this demonstration is by the infliction of an external pain [...] which generally will 'fit the crime' only in the sense of being roughly proportionate to its gravity."[563]

Yet, Burnaby suggests in criticism of Augustine, by applying a legal view to the divine, God becomes the executor of a code which he can protect against frequent violation only through the application of external sanctions.[564] In talking about the existence of evil from Roman justice theory and God the Creator, Burnaby says that, "in this matter Augustine does not come beyond the occasional approach, the momentary glimpse"[565] of the "true meaning" of suffering. The true meaning can be understood when consistently viewed from the perspective of redemption. For Burnaby, the notion of God's love (prominent as it is elsewhere in Augustine) is lacking in his account of physical illness and suffering. Not allowing himself to think out the implications of Christ's suffering, Augustine "rested in a view of suffering, which the revelation of God in Christ has made untenable."[566]

Against Burnaby's critique, Stanley Hauerwas argued in *Naming the Silences* (a book on God, medicine, and human suffering) that suffering for Augustine is a *practical* challenge to his faith, requiring a *practical* response. Ultimately, it is *not* a metaphysical question requiring an abstract answer as it is for Paneloux and Burnaby.[567] Augustine's attempt to make sense of evil cannot be taken as an isolated attempt at logical explanation, Hauerwas says. It is not a theoretical account of the origin of evil and disease in isolation from the overall goal of Christian existence which is the attainment of blessedness.[568]

It would represent an unduly narrow reading of Augustine if his account of evil were taken as an attempt of logical explanation in isolation of God's redemptive action. For Augustine, an understanding of evil and of punishment could not be reached without knowing first of God's restoring and redeeming grace. Opposing joy, suffering for Augustine in the first place appears as a practical challenge to his faith requiring a response.[569] In *The Confessions*, Augustine responds with praise of God to the experience of pain,[570] for God gave him the tools for dealing with his suffering – for instance, the ability to be *patient*.[571]

According to Hauerwas, for Augustine to reflect upon the origin of evil is never a theoretical enterprise, which may call into question the possibility of an omnipotent God.[572] After his conversion to Christianity, the divine love, omnipotence and justice are beyond doubt and require a response of praise under all circumstances, for they exceed all human love and justice. Augustine looked for the

---

563 Burnaby, *Amor Dei,* 212.
564 Ibid., 213.
565 Ibid., 205.
566 Ibid., 206.
567 Hauerwas, *Naming the Silences,* 51.
568 Ibid., 50–53.
569 Ibid., 51.
570 Augustine, *Confessions,* I/i/1.
571 Cf. Rom 8:24–25.
572 Hauerwas, *Naming the Silences,* 51.

conversion of people's hearts, which makes them belong to the community of humans and God, a "community of care"[573] for each other. In this community, Hauerwas concludes, the terror of disease will be absorbed.[574] For him, Augustine's view of disease as punishment of sin is not a theoretical answer to the question of the origin of evil in isolation from his concern with God's love for humanity. Augustine's message remains, "Christ had come as a saviour."[575]

4.5 HEALTH OF THE BODY, DIVINE, AND MEDICAL HEALING

"Christ had come as a saviour."[576] This is, indeed, the overall context of Augustine's reflection on physical disease, health, and healing. He is not interested in a definition of disease or health but in their meaning: what it means for humans to be healthy. His starting point is that health belongs to the history of human salvation; salvation understood not as "an ordered progression towards a distant goal, but a sustained miracle of divine initiative; confidence in human resources, moral and intellectual, is the chief of the obstacles man can place in its way."[577] Bodily health is a gift of grace to be appreciated and desired for the sake of the goodness of its giver.

Augustine's interpretation of physical health as a sign of God's love is most apparent when he talks about the sacrament of baptism, divine intercession in response to prayers and the virtue of patience. Whilst underlining the importance of God's intervention for bodily health, Augustine recommended at the same time medical knowledge and treatment. Yet he did so in the firm belief that natural knowledge of the medical kind had its origin in God's goodness and in his will for salvation.

> "Even the health of the body [...], if you wish to trace things to their cause, can only be explained as coming from God, to whom we must attribute both the being and well-being of all things."[578]

4.5.1 The body and divine healing

Physical health may be restored "in Christ's name either by his sacrament, or by the prayers."[579] Augustine distinguishes two kinds of divine healing: (1) sacramental healing in the waters of baptism, and (2) divine intercession in response to prayer.

---

573 Hauerwas, *Naming the Silences*, 53.
574 Ibid.
575 Brown, *Augustine*, 394.
576 Ibid.
577 Markus, *Sacred and Secular*, XVIII, 22.
578 Augustine, *Way of Life*, 28/55.
579 Augustine, *City of God*, XXII/8.

(1) Baptism, for Augustine, means first of all the forgiveness of sins and the healing of the diseased soul through Christ the physician. Yet on the basis of the body-soul union the renewal of the "old broken self" that begins with baptism includes the renewal of a broken body and might manifest itself in the relief of concrete afflictions: examples show that the new life of the baptised often includes the relief of (even chronic) bodily suffering.

Augustine knew of a man who witnessed to having been cured at baptism not only of paralysis but also of a serious hernia: "He came up from the font of rebirth free from both distressing conditions, as if there had never been anything physically wrong with him."[580] Further, a physician, who suffered from gout, gave his name for baptism. Despite a demonic visitation and consequent increase of pain the night before his admittance into the Church[581] the man pursued his baptism as he had vowed. In the "bath of rebirth,"[582] he was "there and then not only relieved of the pain, which had been unwontedly excruciating, but was completely free from the gout from then onwards, never suffering any pain in his feet for the rest of a long life."[583]

(2) Bodily health is a *temporal* good. Humans cannot be said to be forever healthy but will always undergo alternating periods of health and disease. Temporal goods are not to be despised, as they are helpful for humans on their pilgrimage towards eternal happiness without being the pilgrimage's sole goal. Yet it is appropriate for humans to seek temporal goods, as they may be useful for their journey. It is even appropriate to pray to be granted goods such as health or friendships.

This is the context in which Augustine speaks about people approaching God in prayer and asking for the relief of physical pain and the gift of health. Petitionary prayer is concerned with physical ailments that befall humans, sinners, godless creatures, and mortals.[584] It ranges from a cry for divine mercy for oneself (*deprecatio*) as well as on behalf of others (*intercessio*) to an invitation to God (*invocatio*) into oneself.[585] A *deprecatio* or *intercessio* can be a "tearful prayer for pardon from repentant sinners"[586] which arises out of the grievousness of the human condition. Humans turn to Christ in prayer (either for their own or others' benefit). Christ intercedes for them.

> "*The Word was made flesh, and dwelt among us* (Jan 1:14). There you have both the majesty to which you pray, and the humanity that can pray for you. Referring even to the time after his resurrection, the apostle Paul said of Christ, *He is at God's right hand and intercedes for us* (Rom 8:34)."[587]

---

580 Augustine, *City of God*, XXII/8.
581 Ibid.
582 Titus 3:5
583 Augustine, *City of God*, XXII/8.
584 Augustine, *Ex 2 of Ps* XXIX/1.
585 Weaver, "Prayer", 671.
586 Augustine, *Ex of Ps* XVII/9.
587 Augustine, *Ex 2 of Ps* XXIX/1.

The mediator was innocent but nonetheless weak, "so that he might unite you to God by virtue of his spinelessness, and might draw you near to him by being weak."[588] He carried the wounds of humanity, in order to cure humanity's wounds.[589]

In book 22 of the *City of God* Augustine publishes over twenty examples of effective healing through prayer, baptism as well as exorcism out of a concern "that they should not pass into oblivion, unnoticed by the people in general."[590] For instance, Innocentius, a friend of Augustine and counsellor of the vice-prefecture at Carthage, had unsuccessfully undergone medical treatment for fistu-lae. The moment had come that his torments

> "Had so unnerved him that he felt sure that he was destined to perish under the surgeon's hands. The others tried to reassure him, and urged him to trust in God, and submit to God's will like a man."[591]

When Innocentius' visitors, Augustine amongst them, knelt down for prayer,

> "Innocentius hurled himself forward, as if someone had pushed him flat on his face; and he began to pray. It is beyond the power of words to express the manner of his prayer, his passion, his agitation, his flood of tears, his groans, and the sobs which shook his whole frame and almost stifled his breath."[592]

The next morning when the surgeon arrived to examine the fistula of concern, he found it firmly cicatrised.

Augustine himself, while still an unbeliever, experienced the power of his mother's *intercessio* when he fell ill from fevers at his arrival in Rome. The fever became worse, "and I was on my way out and dying."[593] Yet God heard his mother's prayers and Augustine recovered to full bodily health. "Where she was, you heard her, and where I was, you had mercy on me so that I recovered the health of my body."[594]

At another time, during his vacation at Cassiacium and still before his baptism, Augustine experiences the "miraculous rapidity"[595] with which he was healed after putting trust in God. He recalls how God tortured him with toothache, "and when it became so bad that I lost the power to speak, it came into my heart to beg all my friends present to pray for me to you, God of health of both soul and body."[596] As soon as his friends fell on their knees in prayer, the pain vanished. "But what agony it was, and how instantly it disappeared!"[597]

---

588 Augustine, *Ex 2 of Ps* XXIX/1.
589 Ibid., XXIX/12.
590 Augustine, *City of God*, XXII/8.
591 Ibid.
592 Ibid.
593 Augustine, *Confessions*, V/ix/16.
594 Ibid.
595 Ibid., IX/iv/12.
596 Ibid.
597 Ibid.

4.5.2 The body and medical healing

Now, taking into account Augustine's view of physical disease as a punishment
for sin, and his emphasis on divine healing, can it be appropriate and in accordance with God's will to use medical knowledge for bodily healing? Or are humans
trying to evade God's justice where they have recourse to medicine? Would it not
be more appropriate to focus on confession, repentance, prayer for God's mercy,
and the healing power of the sacraments alone? Five aspects can be distinguished
in Augustine's account of bodily health and appropriate healing responses: (1)
Bodily health reflects the goodness of the created body. (2) It is a *particular* aspect of *general* well-being; it is nothing but "an interim step towards [...] a better
and more certain health"[598] – the health of the whole person. (3) Both being (*that*
humans exist) and well-being (*how* humans exist) have their cause in God. That
humans live is due to the one who created life; that they live happily, healthily, or
joyfully is due to the one who causes happiness, health or joy: to God "we must
attribute both the being and well-being of all things."[599] (4) Temporal health, as
well as happiness and joy, reflect eternal health, and happiness, which is granted
to the believer in the fullness of his or her salvation. Temporal health at the same
time may be a sign of God's restoring grace already present in this world. (5)
Medicine may be an effective means of healing. Yet it is not the only means of
healing: God is known to heal through (i) baptism and (ii) prayer – ways of healing which are indicative of the restoration of physical health in the order of salvation.

When medicine is viewed in the context of salvation, it is seen as co-operating
with God's love for individual people. It takes seriously their stories of being created, restored, and redeemed, and it takes seriously all members of humanity as
interdependent in their movement towards God. Whilst praising the gift of patience, which allows humans to bear pain and physical suffering, and the gifts of
prayer and sacramental healing, Augustine does not dismiss the good of medical
healing which seeks to eliminate pain and suffering. In the *City of God* he lists
medicine or "all the medical resources for preserving and restoring health"[600]
amongst the "important arts discovered and developed by human genius."[601] He
sees in medicine the divine power of love dwelling within the created mind. He
reminds his readers that he is speaking "of the natural abilities of the human mind,
the chief ornament of this mortal life, without reference to the faith or to the way
of truth, by which man attains to the life eternal."[602] Yet both reason and understanding are gifts of God's grace.[603]

Bodily health can be restored through medicine, Augustine says – an approval
of the medical art as operative of God's mercy, which biographical examples con-

---

598 Augustine, *Confessions,* V/x/18.
599 Augustine, *Way of Life,* 28/55.
600 Augustine, *City of God,* XXII/24.
601 Ibid.
602 Augustine, *City of God,* XXII/24.
603 Augustine, *Confessions,* V/iii/4; V/iii/5.

firm. Both G. Bardy in his article *Saint Augustine et les medicines* and J. Courtès in *Saint Augustin et la médecine* detail how Augustine went to see doctors when ill and that, too, he was friends with doctors. Augustine said of himself that he had read many scientific books and emphasised that they were still alive in his memory.[604]

M.E. Keenan reaches the same conclusion in her study on *The Life and Times of St. Augustine as Revealed in His Letters*. She says,

"In all probability the writings of Celsus and the elder Pliny were familiar to him. The prominent physician Vindicianus, a personal friend of Augustine's, was the author of certain medical treatises, and it is not unlikely that these also were known to him. Augustine calls upon the authority of medical men in confirmation of his teaching of the interaction of mind and body."[605]

The restoration of bodily health through medical knowledge needs to be attributed to God; it is God's grace and mercy working in members of the medical profession. It is his love being present in the world, working mercifully on sinners and making use of the good material world. It is a blessing, with which God's goodness has filled human misery on earth.[606] However, humans need to understand that above all it is their spiritual soundness which is of highest importance for their salvation: they should always seek for God's remedies for their soul's illness in the first place.

"It is one thing to cure physical diseases and heal wounds which few men are competent to do [...] but a great number and variety of spiritual maladies are cured only by an extraordinary and ineffable remedy. And if this medicine were not sent to the people of God, there would be no hope of salvation, so unrestrainedly so they continue to sin."[607]

Whilst recognising health of the body, Augustine emphasises the predominance of health as a spiritual phenomenon. This view originates in his *hierarchical* view of the body-soul union with the soul not only animating but above all dominating the body.

4.6 HEALTH OF THE SOUL IN THE CONTEXT OF REDEMPTION

Augustine reflects on disease, death and health both of body and soul from within his vision of human life as integrating the natural, personal, spiritual, and social. Human life in body and soul is the sphere where the presence of God's love may be recognised and responded to. If taken on its own, his account of disease and health does not differ substantially from that of Tatian, Tertullian, or Basil the Great. Augustine, too, accounted for interplay of nature and demons[608] whilst at the same time acknowledging natural causes of disease. Yet his originality lies

---

604 Augustine, *Confessions*, V/iii/3; V/iii/6.
605 Keenan, *Life and Times of St. Augustine*, 24.
606 Augustine, *City of God*, XXII/24.
607 Augustine, *Way of Life*, 28/55.
608 See amongst many other passages on demon possession: Augustine, *City of God*, XXII/8.

with his synoptic anthropology, and above all his interpretation of the soul and the soul's health in the context of the *imago Dei*.

The *imago Dei*, which is located in the specifically human part of the soul and is therefore intrinsic to all human life, indicates the relationship of love between the Creator and the creature as inalienable and intrinsic and as the foundation both of human individuality and sociability. *In being in the image,* humans are at all times addressed by, and capable of relationship to, God. Where they are addressed by God, they are addressed as this particular person: you or me. In this sense, *imago Dei* is foundational of human particularity, individuality, or personhood. However, humans are unable to see their own possibility for relationship due to the discolouring of the image after the Fall. They are unable to realise how their own particularity stems from their relationship to God, and how this relationship connects them with their fellow humans in a relationship of love. The failure to relate to God leads to diseases of the soul, Augustine says. *In becoming the image,* humans move towards the future state of blessedness and of realisation of this relationship, and of goodness. Augustine's reading of the *imago Dei* means for the human soul that it is historical, dynamic, prolepsis, and relational: that which *is* and that which *is not yet*, that which *is* and that which it is moving towards. That which is, is always in relation to God, one self, and the other. That *which is* includes the possibility of disease as of health whereas the soul's health always indicates and anticipates that *which is not yet*.

Augustine's ability to view the health of the soul as the higher good without denying the good of bodily health allows for his recognition of medicine. At the same time, it draws boundaries to medicine's practice. Both claims will be taken up in chapter six.

4.6.1 Health of the soul as higher good

The natural body cannot live of itself but depends in its growth and health upon the good life of the soul, which draws goodness and life energy from its relationship with God. Due to this union, the two kinds of health (and disease) can be neither separated (for humans are the union of body and soul) nor do they need to occur at the same time (for the union is impaired). In other words, humans may be healthy in their souls though obviously showing symptoms of bodily disease.

A rightly ordered relationship to God causes the soul's health. In a letter to his brother Profuturus, Augustine distinguishes both kinds of health where he says,

> "In spirit, as far as it pleases the Lord, and as He deigns to give me strength, I am well, but in body, I am in bed, for I can neither walk nor stand nor sit because of the pain and swelling of haemorrhoids and chafing."[609]

Physically, he suffers and bears the pain of haemorrhoids and chafing, yet at the same time he is well in spirit, for his relationship to God is rightly ordered. And he continues, "Even so, since it pleases the Lord, what else is to be said but that I

---

609 Augustine, *Letter to Profuturus*, 169.

am well?"[610] In accordance with the hierarchy of inner and outer man, or soul over body, Augustine's concludes that spiritual health determines one's overall well-being.

As a small boy Augustine recovered quickly and suddenly from a chest infection. Whilst having regained health in his body, he had not yet received "health of the soul"[611] as his baptism was delayed "on the assumption that, if I lived, I would be sure to soil myself; and after that solemn washing the guilt would be greater and more dangerous if then defiled with sins."[612] Only the sacrament of baptism could have healed his soul and protected him from further illness, Augustine says. On another occasion, when ill in Rome as a young man, Augustine recovered from fever but still remained sick in his sacrilegious heart, "For though in such great danger, I had no desire for your baptism."[613]

Both occasions are contrasted by his lung condition in Milan. This time, the disease was almost met with pleasure by the newly converted as he knew that time-off would enable him to devote himself more fully to God.[614] Despite his bodily illness, he felt to be firmly on his way to spiritual health and therefore inner peace, of which his baptism was the beginning.

When Augustine says that the human soul is diseased, he does not think of mental diseases in the medical sense even though he often uses terms such as disease, illness, and also sleep[615] and death[616] that pertain to the natural sphere. He thinks of the diseased soul in terms of its discoloured-ness – its inability to see God's image clearly, and to seek his love, goodness, wisdom, and truth as ends of action.

Spiritual healing is the life-long process of restoring the image, of orientation of actions towards God. Even though full healing cannot be obtained in the present time, it needs to be striven for, firstly in remitting the cause in baptism, and secondly in orienting the affections aright towards.

> "By believing, I could have been healed. My mind's eye thus purified would have been directed in some degree towards your truth which abides for ever and is indefectible."[617]

Whilst Augustine displays a balanced view of the importance of temporal things (they are good, for they are part of the creation of a good Creator) he admonishes his readers that their soul's eyes, their inner eyes, must always be fixed on eternal things, which are placed above nature, and lead to everlasting happiness.
A part of our reasonable attention, that is, a part of this same mind must be directed to the use of changeable and corporeal things, without which this life does

---

610 Augustine, *Letter to Profuturus*, 169.
611 Augustine, *Confessions*, I/xi/18.
612 Ibid., I/xi/17.
613 Ibid., V/ix/16.
614 Ibid., IX/ii/4.
615 Augustine, *Ex. of Ps.*, XXXVII/III/3. It is a metaphor that evokes the scene in the garden of Gethsemane, where the disciples, overcome by sleep, fall victims to the weakness of their minds and the temptations of their bodies.
616 Augustine, *Confessions*, VI/i/1; VI/iv/6.
617 Augustine, *Confessions*, VI/iv/6.

not continue, not in order that we may be conformed to this world by placing our final end in such goods and in directing our desire for happiness towards them, but that whatever we do in the use of temporal things under the guidance of reason, we do it with our gaze fixed on the eternal things which we are to obtain, passing quickly by the former, but clinging to the latter.[618]

Augustine's hierarchical view of health of body and soul has its origin in his understanding of the body-soul union. As has been analysed earlier, against Neo-Platonist idealism (which identifies the *truly* human with the immaterial soul) and Manichean dualism (which relates the body to the kingdom of darkness) Augustine explicated the union of body and soul from the perspective of incarnation and resurrection. The incarnation of Christ shows first, the union of body and soul in humans, second, the precedence of soul over body and, third, the subordination of both to God's word. The resurrection embraces the whole being "and therefore the body must also, by glorious resurrection, be taken up into eternity."[619] Where the soul speaks to the body from the perspective of its union, it speaks from its position of superiority: the body, and the knowledge that accompanies it, needs to be subordinated to the soul with its distinct, *inward* knowledge of God's love. For Augustine, the superiority of the soul within the body-soul union explains the priority of health of the soul.[620]

4.6.2 Baptism, scripture and the healing of the soul

Like Tertullian, Augustine thought the true relationship between the Creator and the creature could only be restored through baptism. The sacrament of baptism is a remedy[621] and one that ought to be sought for from the earliest age possible. Referring to physical illness, he states that nobody would dare to say when the health of the body is at stake "'let him get worse. He is not yet cured'."[622] Augustine's argument in favour of infant baptism is based upon his understanding of the anabaptised state as one of spiritual illness. Baptism means restoration of the image of God in humans, which is the beginning of the healing of the soul. From baptism onwards, all future spiritual health or illness, the soul's "safety",[623] lies in God's keeping alone.

The removal of inherited sin in baptism does not entail spiritual health once and for all on part of the newly baptised. It is one thing to heal by removing the primal cause of illness and it is another to heal by removing the actual effects of this original sin, namely human concupiscence, which might lead to further illness even in the life of a baptised. The renewal of the *imago*, the healing of the effects of the original sin, is a continuous process.

---

618 Augustine, *Trinity*, XII/12/17.
619 Marrou, *Resurrection and Human Values*, 16.
620 Augustine, *City of God*, XXII/24.
621 Augustine, *Confessions*, IX/iv/8.
622 Ibid., I/xi.
623 Augustine, *Confessions*, I/xi.

"Just as it is one thing to be free from fevers, and another thing to recover from the weakness which has resulted from the fevers; and, similarly, just as it is one thing to remove a spear that has been driven into the body, and another thing to heal the wound that has been made by it through the treatment that follows, so the first step in a cure is to remove the cause of the disease, which is done through the remission of all sins; the second is to heal the disease itself, which is done gradually by making progress in the renewal of this image."[624]

Only if the image of Christ has stamped and moulded the soul (which is what happens in the sacrament of baptism) can the defilement of sinful desires such as envy or greed be reduced. Augustine describes his anabaptised soul as "sick and weak": the image of God inside him was a discoloured, unfinished image – "unmoulded clay".[625] "Formless it [the soul] was prey to every wandering desire, graceless, it was corrupted in concupiscence, lacking Christ, it was in need of salvation."[626]

Where the image of God is blurred and discoloured, as is the case after the Fall and before baptism, the soul is cut off from God's love and abundant goodness, and, too, from the happiness, which only a moral life under the rule of charity can provide. All areas of the anabaptised life reflect the soul's illness. An anabaptised will seek his goods in the external realm and seek with bodily eyes in the light of the sun.[627] Instead the only illuminating light for Augustine is the eternal light of God's wisdom which humans are enabled to discern having gone through the cleansing water of baptism. However, man's full renewal to the image of God or his rebirth into a new life moulded in Christ is not a sudden and immediate conquest of the old nature of Adam.

Spiritual healing, like the restoration of the *imago*, is a gradual process, which takes place during one's lifetime; it is a process helped by drinking from the potion of Scripture, particularly the psalms. "Every sickness of the soul has in Scripture its proper remedy. Let him then whose sickness is of that kind [...] drink this psalm."[628] In the sixth book of the *Confessions* Augustine accounts for the healing influence of Ambrose's teaching of the Scriptures.[629] In the tenth book of the *Confessions*, he recalls "how I cried out to you in those psalms, and how kindled my love for you! Also I was fired by an enthusiasm to recite them, were it possible, to the entire world in protest against the pride of the human race."[630]

The psalms are an antidote for sin; they lead to the cure of spiritual diseases.[631] Reading the psalms, Augustine sees himself in a mirror glass, which reflects his own ill condition. They not only evoke the memories of his former life but also make him re-experience the pain he felt when he was separated from God's love, and hence became diseased in his soul. Augustine's recollection of his misery, provoked by the mirror of the psalms, is meant to serve as a warning to

---

624 Eijkenbloom, *Christus Medicus Motief*, 223; Augustine, *Trinity*, XIV/17/23.
625 Augustine, *Confessions*, I/xi.
626 Rigby, *Original Sin*, 55.
627 Augustine, *Confessions*, IX/iv/9.
628 Augustine, *Ex. of Ps.*, XXXVII/I/2.
629 Augustine, *Confessions*, VI/i/1.
630 Ibid., IX/iv/8.
631 Ibid.

those who are not yet following the God's path. In this, it is therapeutic in character. In Augustine's own words,

> "As I heard the Psalms, I trembled at words spoken to people such as I recalled myself to have been. For in the fantasies, which I had taken for truth, there was vanity and deceit. In the pain felt at my memory of it, I often cried out loud and strong. I wish I could have been heard by those who even now still love vanity and seek after a lie."[632]

Augustine ends the account of his reading of the psalms by emphasising the miraculous rapidity with which God's mercy brings relief.[633] The psalms mirror actual illness of the soul; they serve as diagnosis and remedy. Explaining the diagnostic properties of the psalms in Augustine's thought, M. Fiedrowicz pays particular tribute to their poetic character, because of which "experiences which were originally individual and personal, concrete and unique, attain universal and timeless validity"[634] thus permitting individual appropriation. In this sense, Augustine remarked about a psalm,

> "It grieves with you, and asks questions with you, but not because it does know you. Rather does it ask you the question to which it knows the answer, so that in it you may find what you did not know. [...] The psalm, and indeed the Spirit of God, though knowing everything, asks questions with you, as though giving expression to your own words."[635]

To look into the bright mirror glass of the psalms is the first step towards healing. In a next step however, one has to assimilate oneself to the inspired words of the psalm, wherein then consists the healing of the soul's illness. As Augustine puts it, "the psalm took on your words, now you take on the words of the psalm."[636] Baptism is the beginning of the process of restoration of the soul's health; prayer, scripture and the psalms help on the way; they allow humans to understand God, and God's love, as the end and guiding principle of all human action.

4.6.3 Concluding remarks

The preceding reflection on Augustine's view of the soul's health showed that the knowledge of God situated inwardly in the human soul needs to come prior to the knowledge of physiological processes: only the revelation of love can lead to everlasting, hence, true happiness. Whilst emphasising the precedence of the soul's distinct knowledge, Augustine is adamant that natural knowledge, the knowledge of "changeable and corporeal things," is also given its due. Humans are bodies, that is, natural, temporal and corporeal beings. As bodies, humans benefit from arts that observe the natural world to which their bodies belong.

With reference to the body-soul union, Augustine's theology acknowledges the natural reality of the body and medicine's natural knowledge. However, rea-

---

632 Augustine, *Confessions*, IX/iv/9.
633 Ibid., IX/iv/12.
634 Fiedrowicz, Introduction to Augustine's *Expositions of the Psalms*, 38.
635 Augustine, *Ex. of Ps.*, XCIII/9.
636 Ibid., XCIII/27.

sonable knowledge can never replace revealed knowledge as it cannot provide the health of the soul, which is the restoration of the image of God, a process which will lead to full happiness. Augustine recognises "temporal things" concerned with nature yet he values higher "eternal things" concerned with the desire for everlasting happiness. Whilst the former demand attention, as "our life does not continue" without them, humans need to cling to the latter as it is here only that they may find true joy and happiness.

As the life of the human being is lived in the union of body and soul, the recognition of the body includes at all times the dimension of reality that surpasses mere bodily functioning: the soul, or socio-personal and spiritual dimension of life, as Augustine concluded interpreting the doctrine of the *imago Dei*. His view of the body-soul union in combination with the *imago* allowed him to understand the natural body as the *locus* of God's love. In response to this love, the physician is directed to the patient in an attitude of personal care which goes beyond the repair of physical functions.

Seen from the perspective of God's love, which grounds the promise of salvation, health of body and soul is a graciously granted state of being that anticipates complete and full well-being in body and soul. In its relation to God's absolute goodness, human health always is a relative good.

Hence, Augustine's warning that the restoration of (bodily) health can be no absolute moral imperative to which God, too, would have to bow. This is not to say that the curing of physical diseases is not a morally legitimate endeavour: God's care for humanity and his promise of fullness of life in the presence of death reveals the art and science of medicine as an essentially legitimate but intrinsically limited means of alleviating pain and restoring health.

Whilst these are the conclusions that may be developed from within the framework of Augustine's anthropology, a more detailed exploration is still required of how such a theologically grounded integrative anthropology may frame the understanding of health and medical healing in today's context. This is, then, the purpose of the dialogue with contemporary philosophy in the following chapter.

5. CONCEPTUALISING HEALTH (3): THE ANGLO-AMERICAN PHILOSOPHICAL DEBATE

In 1974, an inaugural transdisciplinary symposium on philosophy and medicine was held in Galveston, Texas, USA. It set the agenda for the field of the philosophy of medicine, and was the starting point for the Anglo-American debate on how to understand the concepts of health and disease in the clinical context. The meeting gathered philosophers with an interest in medicine, the "active philosophy of man,"[637] and members of the medical profession with an interest in philosophical inquiry into medical concepts.

Against the background of medicine's significance for individual human existence, society and health policies as well as its rapidly increasing technical capabilities, the aim of the meeting was to investigate, and critically reflect upon, conceptual issues in medicine. The initiators perceived an urgent need to make medicine a philosophically examined profession and to subject all of its presuppositions and axioms to rigorous re-examination. In being an enterprise of studying *and* refashioning the human condition, H. Tristram Engelhardt reflected that medicine had become "the art and science of remaking man according to man's picture of himself, according to his hopes of what he can be."[638] Edmund D. Pellegrino, participant at the conference, physician, and soon-to-be editor of *The Journal of Medicine and Philosophy*, added the warning that "medicine today has the unprecedented capacity to alter profoundly the lives and the behaviour of individuals and society."[639] An uncritical application of the capabilities of medicine would present an ever-present danger for society.[640]

Notwithstanding the few outspoken and many silent critics, who considered the role the concepts of health and disease play in medical research and clinical practice to be overestimated, initiators and participants of the 1974 symposium in Galveston (and its present day followers) were convinced that above all it is the immediate anthropological, ethical, social and political relevance of these concepts that justifies ongoing and thorough reflection and requires a broad philosophical framework of interpretation. On the basis of a growing recognition of the sociology and philosophy of medical knowledge, and perhaps also under the influence of Michel Foucault's analysis of the clinic/laboratory dialectic and Georges Canguilhem's linking of the relation between health and disease to the requirements of institutional power,[641] Anglo-American scholars started to chal-

---

637 Engelhardt, "Introduction", in: Engelhardt/Spicker: *Evaluation and Explanation*, 5.
638 Ibid., 4.
639 Pellegrino, "Roundtable discussion", in: Engelhardt/Spicker: *Evaluation and Explanation*, 230.
640 Ibid.
641 English translations of both works were available in the mid-1970s.

lenge the dominant positivist ideology of medicine, which discounted personal and cultural evaluation of physical phenomena.

This chapter focuses on the 1970s–1980s debate for the following three reasons: (1) The 1970s reflections on health and disease led to a philosophical framework which is still largely at work in contemporary health debates. If one seeks to engage with, and penetrate, the public debates as they prevail today, knowledge of the 1970s beginnings and its opposing philosophical positions is foundational. (2) Focusing on the Anglo-American debate allows me to explicate the impact that an *isolated* focus on the body, the individual, or the social context may have on medical practice. The debate centres on functions of body, cultural and social influences or individual ends in a largely exclusive way. It does hardly account for their interplay or interdependence. (3) Unlike 1960s French philosophy, the Anglo-American debate does not explicitly focus on power structures or economic and institutional influences. Clearly, this is a deficiency. However, in the context of the present study, it is precisely the debate's focus on the themes of body, sociability *or* individuality which allows for a dialogue with early Christian and Augustinian approaches to health and healing, which look at health and disease from the perspective of human life in its bodily, social, *and* individual dimension.

I will provide an overview of the debate as it has taken place since the 1970s and will point out some of the directions in which the debate has started to move since the mid-1980s. Not only has it widened geographically, in that it now includes more and more European philosophers, but it is also increasingly heading towards theories that seek to bridge natural-factual and socio-cultural-evaluative aspects in order to serve the practical needs of the concepts of health and disease more appropriately. Italian philosopher Roberto Mordacci, for instance, situates health in the context of both physiological knowledge and a notion of human flourishing which anticipates the experience of full life (plenitude). For him, as for his American colleagues James Lennox and Robert Sade, the understanding one has of the notion of health depends upon the notion of human life as serving a goal (also biologically understood) and a good. However, no unifying philosophical framework is available.

Following on from here, I will turn to a more detailed analysis of the philosophical positions from the 1970s that still dominate today's Anglo-American debate. I will look at the American naturalist philosopher Christopher Boorse, who defines health in terms of the statistically normal. He developed his by now classical account of disease and health in three articles published between 1975 and 1977: "The Distinction between Disease and Illness" (1975), "What a Theory of Mental Health Should Be" (1976), "Health as a Theoretical Concept" (1977). According to Boorse, health can be specified independently of ethical or epistemological reflections; it is a matter of empirical investigation. Whilst giving the concepts of health and disease a clear epistemological status, which is practically useful for disease classifications, this approach reduces the concepts to bodily functionality and fails to recognise the individual dimension of health and disease experience. This has implications for the patient-physician relationship and is crucial where doctors seek not only to *cure* but above all to *care* for their individual patients.

Against Boorse's position, the (then) philosopher of medicine[642] H. Tristram Engelhardt argued in his 1974 article "The Disease of Masturbation: Value and Concept of Disease" for health and disease as value-based concepts established through cultural evaluation. Engelhardt, author and editor of numerous articles, series, and monographs on issues of medical morality and bioethical concerns, most recently from the perspective of Orthodoxy or "traditional Christianity" as he calls it, objected to Boorse's exclusively naturalist account while acknowledging that the concepts of health and disease include empirical bodily parameters. Using the example of the nineteenth century disease of masturbation, he argues for a value-infected and culture-dependent concept of health. His approach allows for deconstructing medical ideologies and is able to appreciate the impact of modern day pluralism on science. However, in focusing on the social and cultural context primarily, Engelhardt fails to explore the horizon of individuality and life-experience, which needs to be taken into account where health care also means the action of taking *care* of the person who suffers.

The individual dimension of human life in relation to health is at the centre of Lennart Nordenfelt's account of health. Nordenfelt's approach is an example of how the debate is moving beyond the geographical boundaries of the Anglo-American world (Nordenfelt lives and works in Sweden) as well as beyond the oppositions of naturalist and evaluative approaches in the 1980s. I will focus on his 1987 monograph *On the Nature of Health. An Action-Theoretic Approach* as well as his 1993 articles "Concepts of Health and their Consequences for Health Care" and "On the Relevance and Importance of the Notion of Disease". For Nordenfelt, health is a state of life which serves the achievement of a human being's vital goals. These goals are the result of individual choices. Their achievement determines happiness. Whilst the advantage of Nordenfelt's interpretation is to allow medicine to include the subjective needs and desires of the patient, the question remains how a common (social, cultural, political or indeed natural) underpinning of health can be recognised within such a subjective framework.

Despite their differences, both Lennart Nordenfelt and Christopher Boorse claim second century philosopher and physician Galen to be their intellectual ancestor: indeed, as we have seen, Galen developed an idea of health as the normal or natural state of the body (like Boorse) and situated bodily health within the context of human being's overall striving for welfare (like Nordenfelt). Yet in emphasising *the union* of body and soul, and the corrective influence of reason on the normal state of the rational soul, Galen moved beyond a merely naturalist or individualist account of health, which allowed him to include in his reflection on health a reflection on medical morality.

---

642 H. Tristram Engelhardt now writes as an Orthodox Catholic, see his 2000 monograph on *The Foundations of Christian Bioethics*.

5.1 OVERVIEW OF THE ANGLO-AMERICAN HEALTH DEBATE

"Diseases are to the clinicians what gardens are to gardeners or cars to garage mechanics. These terms are handy to point to a certain area of competence, but the gardener does not need a definition of "garden" to help him decide what to do about plants on a balcony and the garage mechanic does not need a definition of "car" to be able to decide if he should try to fix a lawnmower. [...] To some extent it is true does that the concept of disease plays a certain role in medical thinking, but this role is much smaller than many seem to recognise, and it is particularly small in sophisticated medical thinking."[643]

Is there a *concept* of disease (and health) in medicine that can be the object of analysis? Is medicine indeed grounded on the theoretical concept of disease and health? Or does it rather deal in an immediate, practical way with individual experiences of illness such as discomfort and pain on the one hand, and desires, wishes, and (potential) personal benefits on the other? Of what practical relevance is the theoretical, philosophical discussion of the alleged concepts? Instead of sophisticated philosophical definitions, medicine above all requires "crude concepts and rules of thumb"?[644]

These are some of the questions physiologist Germund Hesslow asks in his article "Do We Need a Concept of Disease?" published in volume 14 of the journal *Theoretical Medicine* in 1993. The article is his contribution to the on-going interdisciplinary debate on issues in the epistemology and methodology of medical practice and research. Hesslow thinks

"Some version of what is sometimes called the 'mechanical model' of disease, that is the view that disease is a deviation from some kind of ideal design, is essentially correct and captures quite well what medical scientists and practitioners actually mean by the term 'disease'."[645]

And he continues, "It is striking [...] that the concepts 'disease', 'illness' and 'health' attract very little interest from clinicians or from medical scientists, and are mainly discussed by philosophers, social scientists and public health officials."[646]

For Hesslow, the concept of disease is neither a necessary nor a sufficient tool for deciding who is (or is not) to undergo medical treatment;[647] it is inadequate for defining the scope of medical insurance;[648] it is not necessary for granting special rights to patients;[649] and the concept of mental disease in particular is not necessary for drawing a line between criminal responsibility and irresponsibility.[650] Questioning both the existence and practical relevance of the concept of disease, Hesslow attacks the branch of Anglo-American philosophy that has been concerned for the last thirty years with reflecting on medical methods and concepts.

643 Hesslow, "Concept of Disease", 13.
644 Ibid.
645 Ibid., 3.
646 Ibid.
647 Ibid., 6–8.
648 Ibid., 8–9.
649 Ibid., 9.
650 Ibid., 9–10.

Until the mid-1970s, Anglo-American philosophy paid little attention to medical epistemology and to the role of health and disease in medical practice. In this it differed from French philosophy with Georges Canguilhem[651] and Michel Foucault[652] as its major representatives. Thomas Kuhn's *The Structure of Scientific Revolutions* (1962) and Paul Feyerabend's *Against Method* (1975) in the sociology and philosophy of medical knowledge remained exceptions, which however helped paving the way for a growing appreciation of the role of cultural and social values in the formation of empirical or scientific facts, and for a questioning of science's neutrality and medical authority.

As a possible reason for this initial lack of attention, philosopher Julius Moravcsik suggested in his 1976 article "Ancient and Modern Conceptions of Health and Medicine" (published in the first volume of *The Journal of Medicine and Philosophy*) that "an adequate treatment of the concepts of health and medicine requires the combination of theories in epistemology, philosophy of science, ethics, and metaphysics."[653] He continued, philosophical reflection in the Anglo-American context "has been too fragmentary to deal with something requiring such a concerted effort."[654] Moravcsik concluded that a new philosophical framework of analysis was necessary, one that would move beyond the positivist analytic framework implicit in much of modern medicine. Moravcsik recommended seeking an account of health and disease in interdependence with ethics, metaphysics, and epistemology, hence, giving up the separation of facts and value.

However, until the mid-1980s, philosophical Anglo-American reflection continued to largely take place between two poles: descriptivist or naturalist theories of health, which deny *any* conceptual relation between health and value, were opposed by a value-based or normativist position.

Christopher Boorse was the unquestioned spokesperson of the naturalist concept of health. His is a still prevailing view: Hesslow refers his understanding of disease to the Boors Ian conception.[655] Normativists by contrast argued against naturalists of the Boors Ian type that (a) health becomes normative for medical practice not through the explanatory force of a descriptive concept but *only* or *largely* through evaluation processes and that (b) all evaluation is conditioned and determined by an individual, social or cultural framework, perhaps almost exclusively.[656] Engelhardt's work represents the normativist position.

With Nordenfelt's 1987 *On the Nature of Health. An Action-Theoretic Approach* the Anglo-American health debate began moving beyond the oppositions of naturalist and evaluative approaches. Since the mid-1980s, new approaches and

---

651 Georges Canguilhem, *Le normal et le pathologique*, 1948/1966, transl. 1978.

652 Michel Foucault, *La naissance de la clinique*, 1963, transl. 1975.

653 Moravcsik, "Ancient and Modern Conceptions", 337.

654 Ibid., 338.

655 Hesslow, "Concept of Disease", 3.

656 See also J. Margolis: "The Concept of Disease" (1976); by H. Fabrega: "Concepts of Disease: Logical Features and Social Implications" (1972), "Social and Cultural Perspectives on Disease" (1980); by E. Pellegrino/D. Thomasma: *A Philosophical Basis of Medical Practice: Towards a Philosophy and Ethic of the Healing Professions* (1981).

bridging theories appeared which broadened the initially bi-polar interpretative framework in taking into account experience, ethics, and metaphysics.[657]

K.W.M. Fulford for instance noted in his article "Praxis Makes Perfect" in the 1993 volume of *Theoretical Medicine* that the objective-factual and the subjective-evaluative poles are much more closely related than may seem at first glance. He considers the concept of illness as a bridging concept. He proposes a theory of illness which emphasises the value-laden nature of the *experience* of illness and analyses illness not in terms of goals of actions but in terms of the internal structure of action which can be described objectively. This combination maintains the "objective, empirically-verifiable dimension of the descriptive theories, and the moment of normativity which can only be accounted for through the value-component of the evaluative or normative theories."[658]

In 1997 Katarina Fedoryka attempted to give yet another new framework for the understanding of health "capable of bridging the gap between theory and praxis with internal theoretical consistency, and of yielding a clearly demarcated notion of health as a normative concept."[659] Fedoryka's conceptual framework involves an understanding of value to be "a property of things" and in this as "a peculiar kind of fact."[660] As she explains, "It implies that while there is a distinction between fact and value, this difference is not that of objective existence versus subjective constitution."[661] She places health within the wider framework of an organism's biological flourishing, that is, the pursuit of certain ends. Fedoryka understands, with medical philosopher Stephen Toulmin, the organism *itself* to evaluate the ends it needs to pursue. From this she concludes,

> "There are two significant points here: the first is to identify health as the flourishing or actualisation of a being, and the second is to limit this flourishing to that which is a direct function of nature, not of individual choice."[662]

Furthermore,

> "The objectivist notion of health as the actualisation of a nature allows, through the ideas of function and natural self-actualisation, for a union of the descriptive and the evaluative moments on both the practical and theoretical levels."[663]

In his 1995 article "Health as an Analogical Concept" Thomist philosopher Roberto Mordacci also reaches beyond the traditionally bi-polar debate. He argues that there is a "clear *logical* priority of health."[664] Health, he says, is the "neces-

---

657 See for instance S.K. Toombs: "The Meaning of Illness: a Phenomenological Account of the Different Perspectives of Physician and Patient" (1992); K.W.M. Fulford: "Praxis Makes Perfect: Illness as a Bridge between Biological Concepts of Disease and Social Concepts of Health" (1993); R. Mordacci: "Health as Analogical Concept" (1995); K. Fedoryka: "Health as a Normative Concept: Towards a new Conceptual Framework" (1997).

658 Fedoryka, "Health as a Normative Concept", 144.

659 Ibid.

660 Ibid., 151.

661 Ibid.

662 Ibid., 153.

663 Ibid., 158.

664 Mordacci, "Health as Analogical Concept", 478.

sary condition"[665] for the experience of illness to be *recognised* as such. Health, in contrast to illness, is not lived consciously[666] but is experienced as lack in the presence of illness or the memory thereof. Illness is experienced as the lacking of possibilities, as a loss or absence of certainty, control, freedom, and as isolation from the familiar world.[667] Against the experience of such an unpleasant state, humans are able to experience health as the desired state. Due to this epistemological and experiential priority of illness, health and disease can be considered neither as mere symmetrical opposites nor as entirely independent concepts. Viewed thus, one can neither simply extrapolate a definition of health from a definition of disease, nor can one talk about health *without* talking about disease. The priority of health as a necessary condition "indicates that health is *more original*, even if experienced in an often unexpressed and not clearly conscious way."[668] Crucially, for Mordacci, illness has a narrow meaning whereas health as the experience of the desired state, of *"life as a good"*, is *"an analogical anticipation* of the hoped-for or simply ideal experience which is meant by 'fullness' or 'plenitude' of existence."[669] In this it is a "richer and wider, and therefore more indeterminate"[670] concept. Against this background, for Mordacci, health is intrinsically bound up with the (socially and culturally conditioned) view one has of human life, its goals, and goods of action. It is not based on statistical or natural considerations but is founded on an idea of human flourishing or human welfare.

Human flourishing cannot be understood in a mainly biological sense, as is the case with Fedoryka: for Mordacci the experience of full life is penultimate; it anticipates a hope that can perhaps be explicated only theologically. Mordacci does not spell this out.

The contributions of Fulford, Fedoryka, and Mordacci are exemplary of the Anglo-American debate's moving into a new arena. The initial 1970s debates about the role of values in conceptualising health now more and more extend into reflections about the role of health and disease in conceptualising human life and life goals as well as the wider relations between human individuals and society.[671]

In the following I return to the initial debate. The oppositions that were formulated in the 1970s still frame the present-day debate and remain the reference point of a large part of contemporary discussions in the philosophy of medicine. Focusing on the debate as it has taken place (and is taking place) between Boorse, Engelhardt, and Nordenfelt allows me to explicate the impact that an isolated

---

665 Mordacci, "Health as Analogical Concept", 478.
666 Cf. Gadamer (2000), *Über die Verborgenheit der Gesundheit.*
667 Mordacci, "Health as Analogical Concept", 477.
668 Ibid., 478.
669 Ibid., 476.
670 Ibid., 478.
671 Further examples of the shifting of the debate are the philosopher of science James Lennox and MD Robert Sade for whom the analysis of health depends upon the notion of human life (Cf. Lennox, "Health as an Objective Value" and Sade, "A Theory of Health and Disease" in *The Journal of Medicine and Philosophy*, Vol. 20/5 which is entirely devoted to "Reconceptualising Health and Disease").

focus on the body, or the individual, or the social context may have on medical practice.

5.2 HEALTH AND BODILY FUNCTIONS: CHRISTOPHER BOORSE

For medical physiologists, health is commonly understood as the "normal" state of the body which is the state that aims at homeostasis.[672] Disease in turn is the disruption of homeostasis: it is an "abnormal state" or "the sum of deviations from normal."[673] In this sense, physician-philosopher Leon R. Kass claimed in his 1974 article "Regarding the End of Medicine and the Pursuit of Health" that health is a

> "natural standard or norm – not a moral norm, not a 'value' as opposed to a 'fact', not an obligation, but a state of being that reveals itself in activity as a standard of bodily excellence or fitness, relative to each species and to some extent to individuals, recognisable if not definable, and to some extent attainable."[674]

For Kass, our understanding of health is not fabricated by the choices and goals of particular societies and cultures; it is an omnipresent natural fact. "The fact that some form of medicine is everywhere practiced – whether by medicine men and faith healers or by trained neurosurgeons – is far more significant than the differences in nosology and explanation."[675]

In a similar vein, American philosopher Christopher Boorse defines health as statistically normal, functional ability.[676] Such a definition of health is, he continues, a "medical truism."[677] In his 1975–1977 articles, he defends an objective, purely descriptive account of disease and health – an account which is independent of cultural, social, moral or metaphysical influence. It focuses on the physiological ends of natural bodies. What are these ends? How can one find out about them? For his definition of health, these are two of the questions which Boorse set out to address.

Having looked at Christopher Boorse's understanding of the human body in terms of its species-typical, functional, and goal-oriented design, I turn to his definition of health as statistical normality, whereby normality is understood as performance of functions with at least statistically typical efficiency. Such a definition is useful in establishing disease taxonomies that are applicable across the

---

672 The Guyton/Hall *Textbook of Medical Physiology* proposes homeostasis as the overarching goal of bodily functioning in that it argues, for instance, in favour of reproduction as a homeostatic function. "It does [...] help to maintain static conditions by generating new beings to take the place of those that are dying. This perhaps sounds like a permissive use of the term homeostasis, but it does illustrate that, in the final analysis, essentially all body structures are organised such that they help to maintain the automaticity and continuity of life" (Textbook of Medical Physiology, 4). It goes beyond the scope of this chapter to discuss different interpretations of homeostasis.

673 Riede/Schäfer, *Pathologie*, 7 (my translation).

674 Kass, "Regarding the End of Medicine", 28.

675 Ibid., 24.

676 Boorse, "Health as Theoretical Concept", 555.

677 Ibid., 563.

human species, Boorse rightly claims. Thus, his definition allows for an international (cross-cultural) body of medical knowledge. However, in failing to acknowledge human individuality as intrinsically present in the body, it can only insufficiently answer to the demands of the patient-physician encounter, which is foundational of clinical medicine.

5.2.1 Functional design of the body

Boorse embraces the classical medical tradition as based upon the Platonist view of the natural as the normal.[678] However, he admits to parting with this tradition where he advances the complete separability of empirical facts and value[679] and where he describes *human nature* as the functional design *statistically* shown to be typical of the species *Homo sapiens*. Boorse looks at human beings with an interest in their being *specimens* of the biological species *Homo sapiens*. Like any other animal species, in the course of evolution *Homo sapiens* developed a number of species-specific characteristics both in terms of physical structure and function (structure and function are inter-related). Such species-typical design contributes to the survival both of the individual and the species as a whole. Unlike Plato, Boorse does not interpret *design* intentionally as in humanly designed artefacts: it does not involve positing a maker and the maker's aims. Instead, it is "strictly *analogous* to the mechanical condition of an artefact"[680] in that it involves evolved functions and has in view the functions' purposes.

Boorse's understanding of natural design as functional implies a *teleology*: organ functions are the *end*, goal or final cause of the organ's structures being arranged the way they are.

> "Cells are goal-directed toward metabolism, elimination and mitosis; the heart is goal-directed toward supplying the rest of the body with blood; and the whole organism is goal-directed both to particular activities like eating and moving around and to higher-level goals such as survival and reproduction."[681]

Organ functions and purposes do not presuppose choices but are inherent to nature. They can be read off nature. What emerges as the Boorsian view of natural design is a set of biological or physiological goal-directed functions on the level of the organism's different systems, sub-systems and parts. "The crucial element in the idea of a biological design is the notion of natural function."[682]

Such a view of instrumentality and finality goes back in general to Plato[683] but in this form more closely resembles Aristotle[684] and Galen (*vide supra*). Boorse

---

678 Boorse, "On the Distinction Between Disease and Illness", 58. Cf. also Petersson, "Health in Plato's Thought", 8.
679 Boorse, "Health as Theoretical Concept", 555.
680 Boorse, "On the Distinction Between Disease and Illness", 59 (my italics).
681 Ibid., 57 (my italics).
682 Ibid.
683 Plato, *Republic*, 357b–358a. "In the Platonic world, geometrical and quasi-geometrical form might have been paramount, but a thorough scientific understanding had always to regard

shares with this tradition the "intuition"[685] (as he says) that the natural design with its intrinsic purposes is the norm, hence, is normative for the concepts of health and disease. Yet, he admits departure from this tradition[686] when he pursues the question as to how one learns about these normal purposes or norms. For Boorse, as for the main tradition of *modern* medical physiology, the normal (or species-typical) is a purely *statistical* notion – not a kind of Platonic ideal of health. The normal is that which can be found *empirically* to be the species typical functions on average.[687]

5.2.2 Health as biostatistical normality

For Boorse, health is functioning that can be said *statistically* to be typical of a species. For example, a blood pressure reading of 120/80 mmHg is a common value. Yet, we might say, a person who consistently has a blood pressure reading of 90/70 mmHg can be in good health, too, for the value of 90/70 mmHg represents the particular person's normal blood pressure. Now, by sampling a large number of particular people, an *average normal* and a *range of normal* are determined from which the statistically normal is derived.

A healthy human being functions according to the pattern which is *statistically* typical for the species *Homo sapiens*. Disease is a species atypical diminishment of species typical functional ability. Function statements describe species characteristics not individual characteristics. Boorse points out, "Our species and others are in fact highly uniform in structure and function; otherwise there would be no point to the extreme detail in textbooks of human physiology."[688]

However, Boorse is aware that statistical normality *alone* fails as a necessary or sufficient definition of health.

> "It cannot be necessary because unusual conditions, e.g. type *O* blood or red hair, may be perfectly healthy. It cannot be sufficient because unhealthy conditions may be typical. [...] There are also particular diseases – artherosclerosis, minor lung inflammation, perhaps tooth decay – that are nearly universal."[689]

Statistical normality can only serve as a definition of health if it is understood as *performance of functions* with at least statistically typical *efficiency*.[690] Efficiency can be measured in terms of contribution to the goals of survival and reproduction, which Boorse suggests as primary goals of life (not only human life) on the basis

form as related to – indeed, as correlative with – physiological or quasi-physiological function." (Toulmin, "Nature of the Physician's Understanding", 34).
684 Aristotle, *Metaphysics*, 1013 a 15; *Nicomachean Ethics*, I.7.
685 Boorse, "Health as Theoretical Concept", 554.
686 Ibid., 555.
687 Ibid., 556.
688 Ibid., 557.
689 Ibid., 547.
690 Ibid., 558.

of what appears in physiology texts.[691] Health then is the *statistically* typical causal contribution to the ultimate goals of survival and reproduction.[692]

Homeostasis figures as another primary goal of bodily functioning in physiological literature, yet Boorse does not take it to be an overall goal. He agrees that many aspects of the normal fit Claude Bernard's homeostasis model;[693] yet "homeostasis cannot", he adds, "profitably be viewed as a general model of biological function. Many life functions are not homeostatic unless one stretches the concept to cover every goal-directed process."[694] In this critical evaluation of homeostasis or equilibrium and balance as ultimate goals of the organism, Boorse departs from the Galenic tradition.

In *The Art of Medicine*, Galen defined health as the "*good* mixture of the simple, primary parts, and *good* proportion in the organs, which are composed of these"[695] thus referring back to the teachings of Platonist philosophy as well as Hippocratic medicine,[696] which looked "upon health as a kind of harmony, balance, and order."[697] Galen spoke about the harmony and balance of qualities and humours *qualitatively*, but was unable to define *quantitatively* what he called harmony or equilibrium.

The *quantitative* description, however, is what Boorse is interested in, and it is to this that his statistical understanding of health is directed. He is not interested in the ways in which health is desirable because it points towards, or pertains to, supposed goods such as harmony, balance and order, or even beauty and goodness, but only insofar as "it promotes goals one can justify on independent grounds."[698] For him, these are not goods as such, they do not intimate anything (supposedly) intrinsically desirable, but the basic species typical goals of survival and reproduction.

5.2.3 Concluding remarks

Christopher Boorse advanced a concept of health based on empirical observation and statistical facts about the human species' functioning. His interpretation of health claimed independence not only of metaphysical considerations but also of the particularities of individual choice, of social constructs, cultural values and

---

691 Boorse, "Health as a Theoretical Concept", 556.
692 Ibid., 555/562. However, one might want to ask here whether bodily activity that fails to contribute towards these goals, such as, for instance, masturbation or homosexual intercourse (or indeed any kind of sports) is *per definitionem* diseased functioning (though possibly not experienced as illness).
693 Boorse, "Health as Theoretical Concept", 549.
694 Ibid., 550.
695 Galen, *The Art of Medicine*, 347 (my italics).
696 Hippocrates, *The Nature of Man*, 4. "Health is primarily that state in which these constituent substances are in the correct proportion to each other, both in strength and quantity, and are well mixed."
697 Plato, *Timaeus*, 82a; Petersson, "Health in Plato's Thought", 3–7.
698 Boorse, "On the Distinction Between Disease and Illness", 61.

economic paradigms. Boorse's framework was (and, with modifications, still is) implicit in clinical nosology and disease taxonomies. It eliminates the subjective elements of experiences of health or illness in favour of generalised anatomical or physiological descriptions of what are considered to be objective and neutrally descriptive facts.

Boorse defines health on the basis of his view of natural reality. His is a description anchored in the sphere of nature, where the general laws of physics and mathematics give rise to physiological regularities as well as particularities. Boorse's naturalism, and indeed medicine's naturalism, powerfully gives the natural dimension of human existence its due.

Focusing on the natural functions of the body, Boorse offers an analysis of the body and its state of health which excludes the social, moral or political factors and goals that condition and shape his subject matter. He explicitly rejects ideas of what he calls "positive health" which includes the view that "physicians and mental health workers should actively aid individuals, or communities, in maximising their quality of life and developing their full human potential."[699] Boorse's interpretation of health allows him to limit the scope of clinical medicine to physical and physiological derangements. He does not pursue the question as to whether health also describes, or evaluates, how a woman or man *ought* to live in pursuance of certain goods. His interest is in giving a descriptive account of what humans *are* according to their biological nature. He is careful to avoid prescribing the recipe for an ideal human being.[700] In this, it avoids the fallacy of moral arguments from natural design. Boorse is at pains to avoid giving the notion of health any good-oriented and therefore moral implications, which he considers dangerous in the clinical context: the advocacy of "positive health" raises moral dilemmas about the good human life, which no medical procedure can possibly resolve. He warns,

> "We must avoid confusing empirical questions with deep normative issues about the goals of human life and the role of health professionals in achieving them. The trouble with calling physical or mental or moral excellence "health" is that it tends to unite under one term a value-neutral notion, freedom from disease, with the most controversial of all prescriptions – the recipe for an ideal human being."[701]

Boorse admits that his biostatistical account does not cover structural abnormalities (such as a congenital absence of the appendix which is entirely asymptomatic)[702] or universal genetic diseases (such as the "senile decline of function caused from within")[703] yet considers it a mistake if such problems were taken to invalidate his general approach to health. "Instead they should be viewed as anomalies deserving continued analysis."[704]

---

699 Boorse, "Health as Theoretical Concept", 568.
700 Ibid., 572.
701 Ibid.
702 Ibid., 565.
703 Ibid., 567.
704 Ibid.

Otherwise, the only alternative is the position expressed by H. Tristram Engel-hardt, who views health, Boorse says, as "a vehicle for changing human goals and expectations."[705] Such an account, he argues, is so tolerant that it includes in medical disease inventories of "whatever physicians may come to count as dis-eases" and cannot exclude what they do not count.[706] In contrast to his own model, Engelhardt's account has no explanatory power whatsoever and, what is more, it may involve physicians in unethical or even frivolous endeavours of creating the "ideal human being".

Whilst Boorse's definition of disease and health in biological and functional terms is necessary indeed for the setting up of general disease inventories, it is clearly not sufficient for daily medical practice in that it fails to acknowledge the importance of individual experience and individual interpretations of symptoms as well as socio-cultural factors for the physician-patient interaction.

The vast amount of socio-psychological research that has been conducted on the doctor-patient relationship (Talcott Parsons' 1951 *The Social System* being the classic starting point) cannot be treated here in detail. However, two points shall be mentioned which illustrate the practical limitations of the Boorsian account of health and disease.

(1) The clinical encounter depends on the individual patient's dealing with his or her symptoms of bodily dysfunctioning. Unless the patient considers medical help necessary, it is of no practical relevance whether or not the symptoms he or she has are listed as particular disease symptoms in a disease inventory. In many (perhaps even most) cases, a loss of bodily functions becomes a medical concern only where the patient chooses to make it one by seeking medical advice. Condi-tioned by social, cultural, personal and moral factors, some people may decide to suppress or deny the existence of bodily symptoms even while harbouring (or experiencing) a serious loss of functions. "One can have serious dysfunctional states and diseases and still deny or misinterpret symptoms and thus delay in pre-senting with complaints to physicians."[707]

(2) An exclusively naturalist account of diseases and health with its claims to objectivity does not require the patient *as an individual* (and with the diverging opinions on disease this might entail) to play an active role in the treatment pro-cess. In this, Boorse's account allows for a paternalist model of medicine. It suf-fices for the patient to hand over the dysfunctional body; the physician holds the (epistemological and technical) keys to healing. She starts her work on the basis of her knowledge of functions, laboratory parameters and statistical data; if the patient agrees on her natural analysis, a treatment plan can be worked out, also with the patient's co-operation.

Yet a doctor's data gathering does not involve physical examination and la-boratory parameters alone: for once, it also and always includes verbal and paraverbal communication between two individuals *beyond* the objective descrip-

---

705 Boorse, "Health as a Theoretical Concept", 567.
706 Ibid.
707 Siegler, "Doctor-Patient Encounter", 634.

tion of symptoms. Where patient and physician meet, the patient contributes to the complex diagnostic process through verbal and paraverbal, conscious and subconscious information. The communication between two persons makes the clinical encounter a subjective, personal encounter. To acknowledge the subjective element is indeed crucial for effective treatment. Patients cannot normally name diseases, and formulate a final diagnosis. Nor can they devise therapies: indeed, this knowledge belongs to the domain of the doctor who has received training in the understanding of bodily functions. Here the input of Boorse's theoretical reflection on the concept of disease is important. However, for the encounter to be effective overall (i.e. in the Boorsian sense, as restoring functions effectively), the patient's and the physician's *shared* and *personal* involvement in the diagnostic and following therapeutic process is decisive.

To this H. Tristram Engelhardt would remark that it is equally crucial to understand how such shared and personal involvement in diagnosis and therapy is at all times value-infected and culture-dependent. Even functional-sounding disease definitions can be mere constructs and may result from culturally conditioned evaluation. According to Engelhardt's analysis, successful diagnosis and treatment depends fundamentally on both the physician and the patient subscribing to the same cultural and social interpretation of a particular ontological state or course of bodily activity.

5.3 CULTURAL VALUES AND HEALTH: H. TRISTRAM ENGELHARDT

H. Tristram Engelhardt relates health and disease to the wider goals of human life established not on an individual basis but within a particular societal and cultural context. He has written many articles and monographs on conceptual issues in medicine, most recently from the perspective of Orthodox theology. The analysis in this section mainly draws on his 1974 article "The Disease of Masturbation: Value and the Concept of Disease" published shortly after the afore-mentioned Galveston symposium. Though this article cannot any longer be taken to be typical for Engelhardt's positions as regards disease or indeed human sexuality,[708] it

---

708 In his 2000 monograph *Foundations of Christian Bioethics* Engelhardt views disease as a phenomenon that presents humans not only with natural limitation and bodily finitude but "most significantly with sin and its consequences" (309). He emphasises that by accepting the suffering caused by diseases, which we can ultimately not avoid, "we can give substance to our repentance, abandon pride, and purge the heart from the passions that control us" (315). As for human sexuality, Engelhardt now perceives it as firmly placed "within the history of salvation and the journey to God" (239). It serves the development of the intimate bond between husband and wife, which always needs to be directed towards greater union with God. "All human carnal sexuality and reproduction are to be undertaken within the marriage of one man and one woman, therefore excluding as sinful not just pornography and extramarital sexually evoking circumstances and images, but also masturbation, fornication, adultery, homosexuality, and acts of bestiality" (238). Thus, whilst he refrained from evaluating acts of masturbation in his 1970s article, in his most recent guise Engelhardt presents us with explicit value judgements of *types of sexual activity* – not of the person committing them.

may be taken to be typical for the evaluative understanding of health and disease which opposed a Boorsian kind of naturalism. In his approach to health,[709] Engelhardt never advocates an exclusively evaluative definition; rather, his aim is to draw attention to the *ambiguous nature* of the concepts of health and disease. And this is why his article on masturbation is crucial. The example of masturbation allows Engelhardt to illustrate how the concepts of disease and health always operate on both a descriptive and normative level. Against Boorse's exclusively descriptive account, Engelhardt wants to show that the concepts operate

> "Both as explanatory and evaluatory notions. They describe states of affairs, factual conditions, while at the same time judging them to be good or bad. Health and disease are *normative as well as descriptive*."[710]

Having looked at Engelhardt's analysis of the phenomenon of masturbation classified and treated as a disease in the eighteenth and nineteenth centuries, I will turn to his suspicion that in medicine, as in any other natural science, a moral or aesthetic judgement about an ontological condition comes first. It motivates medical, or scientific, activity. Norms and standards of a particular culture and society determine medical descriptions of physical reality. Against Boorse, descriptions of the body are not neutral descriptions of functions.

Such deconstruction of medical disease classification allows Engelhardt to acknowledge the influence of culture and societal demands on both physicians' and patients' interpretations of disease and health. However, if such an evaluative account of health fails to recognise the reality of the body (which Engelhardt's does *not*), as well as the counterbalancing role of human individuality, the patient risks becoming an object of social engineering. Further, where individuality is not acknowledged sufficiently, patients may fail to experience the personal care which medicine as a science and art should be striving for.

5.3.1 Case study: the disease of masturbation

In Engelhardt's view as present in the 1975 article, medicine does not simply concern itself with understanding, describing, appreciating and treating *the natural* that *is*. It indeed describes and explains, yet where it describes and treats, it is at the same time concerned with *pronouncing*, and bringing about desirable ends and states of goodness that *should be* according to the norms and standards of a particular culture and society. Evaluation enters the enterprise of medical explanation. The example of masturbation shows how medicine's nosology – at work both in research and practice, and in somatically and mentally oriented medicine – is bound up with culturally determined moral judgements. The medical profession translates these judgments into ontological descriptions.

---

709 Cf. Engelhardt's 1975 "The Concepts of Health and Disease".
710 Ibid., 125 (my italics).

"Although vice and virtue are not equivalent to disease and health, they bear a direct relation to these concepts. Insofar as a vice is taken to be a deviation from an ideal of human perfection, or 'well-being', it can be translated into disease language."[711]

The so-called disease of masturbation is not the only example of such translation of moral judgement into ontological language. Engelhardt adds *drapetomania*, another nineteenth century disease of which the symptom was the slave's running away from the slave owner. *Kleptomania* might be added as another such disease, as might also, on another tack, the twentieth century debates on homosexuality, on attention deficit syndrome (ADHD) amongst today's school children or on chronic fatigue syndrome (ME) amongst adults. By contrast, events such as childbirth are not considered to be diseases, even though they involve considerable pain as well as morbidity and mortality.[712] Clearly, forms of social judgement are at work in such disease classifications, Engelhardt says, and continues in his 1975 article on "The Concepts of Health and Disease",

"To call alcoholism, homosexuality, presbyopia, or minor hookworm infestation diseases, involves judgments closely bound to value judgments. Granted, there is a spectrum from broken limbs to colour blindness along which interest in construing a constellation of phenomena as a disease varies. The pain and discomfort of either a broken limb or a schizophrenic break invite immediate medical aid, while issues of colour blindness or dissocial behaviour lie at the other end of the spectrum. But all along the spectrum, *the concept of disease is as much a mode of evaluating as explaining reality.*"[713]

Until the early eighteenth century masturbation was not widely accepted as a disease. Yet by the end of the nineteenth century in a changed cultural setting a broad class of observed signs and symptoms of deranged functions as well as further illnesses, even cases of death were attributed to masturbation as their one causal mechanism. Masturbation was said to be a disease that produced *via* excess and excitation patho-physiological changes in the human body.

"Masturbation was held to be the cause of dyspepsia, constrictions of the urethra, epilepsy, blindness, vertigo, loss of hearing, headache, impotency, loss of memory, irregular action of the heart, general loss of health and strength, rickets, leucorrhoea in women and chronic catarrhal conjunctivitis. Nymphomania was found to arise from masturbation, occurring more commonly in blondes than in brunettes. Further, changes in the external genitalia were attributed to masturbation."[714]

Recommended therapies ranged from dietary to extremely unpleasant surgical procedures, such as vasectomy or castration. The concept of masturbation as a physical disease developed, Engelhardt shows, on the basis of a general moral suspicion that sexual activity was debilitating.[715]

"In the nineteenth century, one was pleased to think that not one bride in a hundred of delicate, educated, sensitive women accepts matrimony from any desire of sexual gratification:

---

711 Engelhardt, "The Disease of Masturbation", 248.
712 Engelhardt, "Concepts of Health and Disease", 139.
713 Ibid. (my italics).
714 Engelhardt, "The Disease of Masturbation", 236.
715 Ibid., 239.

when she thinks of this at all, it is with shrinking, or even with horror, rather than with de-sire."[716]

Against this background, the theoretical framework for the disease of masturbation was not value-free but structured by the life goals and expectations of the times, expressing themselves as moralistic norms, not to mention in this case gender politics.

In the second half of the twentieth century, by contrast, articles were published for the instruction of women *in the use of* masturbation to overcome frigidity or orgasmic dysfunction, now considered as diseases according to the changed outlook on human sexuality. Or, as might be added to Engelhardt's example, the same can be said for twentieth century men, who, too, can suffer from comparable disorders such as premature ejaculation or impotence. Engelhardt's observations seem accurate where he describes sexual activity as now popularly considered a good to be sought for one's overall well-being. Sexuality is no longer the moral evil to be avoided, rather is chastity considered a peculiar psychosomatic disorder. At least in the Western world, Engelhardt remarks, the normative background against which masturbation was to be classified as disease has not only disappeared but has indeed been inverted.[717]

5.3.2 Translation of value judgements into medical concepts

"In explaining the world, one [the scientist] judges what is to be significant or insignificant. For example, mathematical formulae are chosen in terms of elegance and simplicity, though elegance and simplicity are not attributes to be found in the world as such. The problem is even more involved in the case of medicine which judges what the human organism should be (i.e., what counts as 'health') and is thus involved in the entire range of human values."[718]

Both in the case of masturbation as a disease and of chastity as a disorder, social and cultural views, expectations, goals and value judgements structure the description and appreciation of natural reality. Moral suspicions and verdicts precede today's scientific and medical explanation of bodily functioning or dysfunctioning as much as they did in the eighteenth and nineteenth centuries.

From Engelhardt's perspective, variations in the appreciation of natural reality are not due to mere fallacies of scientific method but involve a basic dependence on the logic of scientific discovery and hence upon prior moral evaluations of reality.

"A 'disease entity' operates as a conceptual form organising phenomena in a fashion deemed useful for certain goals. The goals, though, involve choice by man and are not objective facts, data 'given' by nature. They are ideals imputed to nature."[719]

---

716 Engelhardt, "The Disease of Masturbation", 246.
717 Ibid., 247.
718 Ibid., 234.
719 Ibid., 248.

Voluntary human judgement (which takes place in a socially and culturally conditioned context) is translated into disease language. Disease then, for Engelhardt, can be no *intrinsic* evil nor can health be an *intrinsic* good. In calling something disease or health, value is ascribed to certain natural phenomena *a posteriori* according to a choice made by humans. Only when a judgment has been made about the cultural and social value of a particular bodily or mental state of being or activity, can this particular state or activity be organised and labelled as a disease (that is, something to be eradicated) or as health (that is, something to be fostered).

Human goals are dependent upon cultural, social and political context. Evaluation according to these goals always preceded and still precedes medical explanation of nature, Engelhardt says. Crucially, the shift from evaluation to explanation is accompanied by a shift of language "from an explicitly ethical language to a language of natural teleology."[720] As Engelhardt puts it,

> "In shifting to disease language, one no longer speaks in moralistic terms (e.g. 'You are evil'), but one speaks in terms of a deviation from a norm which implies a degree of imperfection (e.g. 'You are deviant')."[721]

In other words, the value-laden language of morality is translated into the supposedly value-neutral language of natural teleology. This act of translation provides modern medicine with the supposedly objective authority of the natural sciences that is required in a political climate of moral pluralism which seeks rational (hence, faith-neutral) authority for its actions.

5.3.3 Concluding remarks

H. Tristram Engelhardt's deconstructionist view as presented in "The Disease of Masturbation" is able "to perform an important iconoclastic function *vis à vis* established medical ideologies"[722] above all *vis à vis* the prevailing claim of the descriptive objectivity and neutrality of science. In questioning the neutrality of scientific explanatory concepts of disease, he also questions the objectivity of natural science and of the factual modes of explanation which Boorse proposed and defended.

Engelhardt analyses the ways in which scientific concepts, thus also the concepts of disease and health, are bound up with larger cultural projects and general life goals, which are preceded by, and include, moral choices and judgments. He acknowledges the impact of human sociability and culture for the understanding of bodily reality, and its gender-specific character. His questioning is not only an epistemological possibility but has ample consequences for clinical practice. Engelhardt acknowledged elsewhere[723] that concepts of disease and health include empirical bodily parameters. He does not deny natural reality, which can be de-

---

720 Engelhardt, "The Disease of Masturbation", 248.
721 Ibid.
722 Khushf, "Reflection on Health and Disease", 465.
723 See Engelhardt (1975), "The Concepts of Health and Disease."

scribed empirically. Yet in his article on masturbation, he illustrates how "the concept of disease has fuzzy borders with moral concepts."[724]

Notwithstanding the valuable contributions Engelhardt makes to the understanding of the ambiguous nature of disease and health and to a physician-patient encounter that recognises the social and cultural dimension of human life and the influence of culture and society on the patient's interpretations of his or her bodily reality, his analysis may create problems in that it may lead to a view which not only (and rightly) denies the *neutrality* of descriptions of natural reality and physiological processes, but which also denies that there *is* natural reality *per se* which is not simply manufactured by humans and a product of the human mind.

Whilst this is *not* Engelhardt's position at the time,[725] in his article on masturbation the description of bodily symptoms results from human (cultural, social, or moral) evaluation processes alone.

What does this mean for the reality of bodily symptoms, and as a consequence, the reality of the body? The problematic consequence of such a claim where taken as exclusive (which Engelhardt did *not*) is that there may be as many human-made bodily realities as there are different cultures, societies, political, and moral systems. Accordingly, there is not one notion of disease or health but as many different diseases and healths as there are different life goals and moral viewpoints in different social and cultural contexts. Then, a cross-cultural body of medical knowledge is plainly impossible.

Yet the neglect of the reality of the natural poses a real danger, perhaps even a tyranny, in the modern biotechnological age Gilbert Meilaender points out in his 1998 monograph *Body, Soul, and Bioethics*. Where nature ceases to be understood as both *real* (as Boorse claimed) and *of value* (against Boorse), where "we have lost touch with the natural history of bodily life,"[726] Meilaender warns, we risk ending up with a view of humans as mere exponents of ideas, as representing a particular cultural or societal status, as persons who *have* certain qualities and capacities such as freedom, autonomy, reason or will, which can be given as well as taken away from them. Where humans do not at a fundamental level attend to the reality of the organic body (let alone to its intrinsic value), bodily persons and their natural states can become the object of voluntaristic social engineering – a

---

724 Engelhardt, "Concepts of Health and Disease, 140.
725 For his more recent views on nature and the human body, see his 2000 monograph *The Foundation of Christian Bioethics*. Here he says that nature is everything created, including the created human body. Yet at the same time, and in addition, it is also natural for man to worship and turn noetically to God, which is an experience that transcends nature (173). However, nature as creation after the Fall is "broken" (174), which makes what is now natural improper and often turned against humans: "The nature of man himself as well as the physical and biological nature that surrounds him is deaf to human purposes, if not hostile to them" (175). Engelhardt here has in mind everything from earthquakes to tornadoes and hurricanes, from conflict and violence to corporeal desires and sexual lust. Whilst Engelhardt questioned the normative character of nature in the 1970s, he now claims broken nature to have become normative. It has its meaning "constituted normatively through this web of desires, including inclinations to evil" (175).
726 Meilaender, *Body, Soul and Bioethics*, 50.

danger which Christopher Boorse realised when he warned against the tyranny of positive health, whilst failing to see that the body is *both* real *and* of value (see also chapter six).

Further, in emphasising cultural and societal influences on human interpretation of natural reality and disease concepts, one may not sufficiently take into account the importance of the *individual* and his or her personal life story and embedded experience of health and disease. Of course, such experience is culturally and socially conditioned (not to mention political and economic influences). Yet the ontological reality of individual human life integrates both *the natural* and *the personal* in its social and cultural dimensions and integrates on this basis *explanation* and *evaluation*. This is Engelhardt's claim in "The Concepts of Health and Disease".

A failure to see this has implications for the patient-physician encounter. As has been shown in the previous section, the individual patient's ability or desire to choose to see a doctor about certain bodily symptoms marks the beginning of the physician-patient encounter, and hence, the beginning of a possible restoration of health. And where the clinical encounter also means the action of taking *care* of the patient, both the initial choice and the encounter that follows cannot be made sense of exclusively in terms of bodily functions or cultural or social influences, but needs to be looked at in the context of the patient's character and personal life-story – which of course is not lived in a cultural and social (or indeed political) vacuum. Where individual agency *as well as* cultural and social components in determining health and disease are taken into account, the patient may have a more active role in determining not only the burden of his or her illness but also the appropriateness of certain kinds of treatments in the context of his or her vision of life and of life's goals.

Engelhardt himself was aware of the importance of individuality for the understanding of health without, however, exploring it further. In "The Concepts of Health and Disease" he states that health is the securing of "the autonomy of the individual from a particular class of restrictions."[727] In this sense, there is only one health, he concludes, "a regulative ideal of autonomy directing the physician to the patient as person, the sufferer of the illness, and the reason for all the concern and activity."[728]

In order to further look at the aspect of human individuality in connection with human agency and life goals in the context of health and disease, I will turn to Lennart Nordenfelt whose account of health is placed within the wider framework of individual action directed at well-being or happiness.

---

727 Engelhardt, "Concepts of Health and Disease", 141.
728 Ibid.

5.4 HEALTH AND THE INDIVIDUAL AGENT: LENNART NORDENFELT

Christopher Boorse wrote his major articles at a time in which the role of culture and society in the formation of empirical facts was being increasingly recognised. Of this development H. Tristram Engelhardt is typical. Engelhardt focuses on the role of values as opposed to natural facts in describing the states of health and disease, and advocates an understanding of health and disease that recognises both their explanatory and evaluative power. However, his focus is more on the evaluation processes within societies rather than the value judgments of individual moral agents independent of their societal context. Engelhardt's analysis also shows that concepts claiming scientific and medical authority can dominate human bodily life rather than serve it.

Lennart Nordenfelt's approach to the concept of health follows the antagonism of the early years, yet attempts to overcome the contradiction of a biostatistical health which claims a place for bodily health separate to social values, and its evaluative counterpart for which H. Tristram Engelhardt came to stand at the time. Nordenfelt places the individual as an agent at the centre of its conceptual analysis, and views it as part of a wider network of social relations. Nordenfelt's is a vision of human life as the life of the "active creature living in a network of social relations."[729] The actions of the individual are always goal directed and a feeling of well-being preconditions any action. Based on this, Nordenfelt understands health as the state of the individual in a societal context in which he or she can achieve their *vital goals*. These are sufficient for the achievement of minimal happiness, so that health is a state that leads to minimal happiness. The individual agent in the context of societies and cultures constantly evaluates both the vital goals and minimal happiness. As a result, there can be as many notions of health as there are individual evaluations of goals. Nordenfelt's individualised account of health allows clinical medicine to centre on the individual's needs and desires. The doctor becomes *the enabler* – the person, who enables the patient to achieve his or her vital goals. Yet such largely subjective interpretation of health does not allow for a shared body of medical knowledge across individuals and cultures and for a generally recognised body of moral medical conduct.

5.4.1 Goal-directed human agency and health

Lennart Nordenfelt's starting point is socio-anthropological. Health as a phenomenon of life does not refer to the body alone, for life is not a mere physiological phenomenon. It involves the human individual as a social agent and his or her ways of acting in society. A human being is not simply assembled parts that form a well-functioning organism but an *acting individual* dependent upon other individuals and their actions. The importance here is Nordenfelt's view of the human being as an *individual* agent and at the same time as a *social* agent. The human

---

729 Nordenfelt, "Concepts of Health and Consequences for Health Care", 279.

individual is a "socially integrated *agent* who performs a great number of daily activities and is involved in many personal and institutional relations."[730]

According to Nordenfelt, human actions are understood to be typically part of an agent's desire to reach certain goals. A number of factors have an impact on the *practical* possibilities of somebody's performing an action. Yet unlike in the Boorsian account, the human ability to perform certain goal-oriented actions does not refer to biological functions primarily, but to the abilities of the human individual *in its cultural and social context*. The ability of an individual for certain actions depends on "a set of standard circumstances"[731] relative to the natural and cultural environment.

> "The decision as to what should count as a standard circumstance for a particular action type is partly influenced by statistical factors, but is mainly determined by the society's profile of goals."[732]

Here, one may detect an influence of Engelhardt's analysis of disease as determined by cultural evaluation processes. Engelhardt's primary concern was with the socio-cultural dimension of illness and the role of moral judgment, that is, the question of the relationship between disease and vice or health and virtue. Yet Nordenfelt is interested less in the ways in which norms and goals are established within societies, but more how the natural, cultural and societal environment *enables* or *hinders* the performance of an individual's goal-directed actions, thus, how the environment allows for the individual's welfare.

In his words,

> "Assume that *G* is a vital goal common to most people in both the societies *S1* and *S2*, and that *G* is much more easily fulfilled in *S1* than in *S2*. The psycho-physical resources needed for realising *G* in *S2* are much greater than in *S1*. To be able to achieve *G* in *S1* is then significantly different from being able to achieve *G* in *S2*. To be healthy in *S1* [...] means then something different from being healthy in *S2*. [...] Observe, however, that strictly speaking this does not mean that the two societies have different *concepts* of health. In both *S1* and *S2* health is defined in the following way: *A* is in health, if, and only if, *A* is, given standard physical and societal circumstances, able to fulfil his vital goals."[733]

Engelhardt's purpose was perhaps polemical, and most certainly iconoclastic. His interest was in exemplary cases, both historical and contemporary, on the basis of which he was able to question and deconstruct the notions of objectivity and value-neutrality in some definitions of health. Nordenfelt's concern is, like Boorse's, more constructive and practical-oriented in that it seeks to find a universally applicable definition of health. In taking into account social and cultural influences on individual human action, Nordenfelt recognises the intrinsic individual and social nature of human existence and avoids the restrictions of a Boorsian kind of biologism. Yet unlike Engelhardt (at least in 1974) he does not neglect the biological dimension of human existence. To this aspect I turn in the next section.

---

730 Nordenfelt, *On the Nature of Health*, 35.
731 Ibid., 49.
732 Ibid.
733 Ibid., 120.

5.4.2 Vital goals, individual happiness, and health

Nordenfelt posits that health does not correlate to all goals but only to what he calls *vital goals*. Nordenfelt modifies two important proposals for a definition of vital goals – namely, "(a) the vital goals of man can be deduced from his basic needs (the need-theory)" and "(b) the vital goals of man are identical with the goals that he himself sets during the course of his life (the subject-goal theory)."[734] He seeks to improve both theories to the effect that "the vital goals of a human being are goals whose fulfilment is necessary and jointly sufficient for the *minimal happiness* of their bearer."[735]

Though health is connected with happiness (for the achievement of vital goals can bring happiness), health is not a necessary or sufficient condition for humans to be happy. One might be healthy and unhappy at the same time, Nordenfelt says, due to on-going war, natural disasters or the like. He leaves undetermined where exactly the level of minimal happiness is to be placed. This is intentional, for happiness cannot be determined statistically or empirically, he says, nor is it merely construed within the frame of societal norms. It depends upon constant *individual* evaluation processes which take place within the frame set by the cultural and social context *en large*. Minimal happiness does not depend *necessarily* on the basic necessities of life such as having food, a sheltered home or economic security, but on a judgment made by the individual agent or by external observers, for instance in the case of infants or the mentally disabled. Nordenfelt is prepared to include biological goals and basic necessities such as survival and reproduction only as far as *the individual agent considers them necessary* for his or her minimal happiness.

> "The criterion of whether a certain state of affairs is a vital goal of A's is whether this state is necessary for the minimal intensity, frequency, richness and duration of A's feelings of happiness. If the question concerns A's health or A's vital goals the evaluation should concern A's happiness and nothing else."[736]

Whilst Nordenfelt recognises that each human individual is part of a network of relations (and in this is a *social* individual), and that the cultural and societal environment conditions and contextualises individual agency, his account of health is fundamentally *individualised* in that the definition of health depends on the agent's individual feelings, desires, ambitions, abilities, and goals. The vital goal of minimal happiness is filled with content according to an autonomous agent's individual hierarchy of goals: society and social relations form the context in which these goals can or cannot be achieved. The value and definition of health is based on individual decision making; such decision-making is, of course, framed, enabled, and at times limited by the natural and social context in which human action takes place. Yet whilst *bios* and society as the context of action might encourage or hinder certain actions, they cannot determine the ends and ways of

---

734 Nordenfelt, *On the Nature of Health,* xv.
735 Ibid.
736 Ibid., 91.

human activity, Nordenfelt argues. Ultimately, it is the individual agent who decides on his or her level of minimal happiness according to whatever he or she holds to be important goals in life.[737] For Nordenfelt, then, there are as many possible healths, not as there are cultural norms, but as there are individual desires, feelings or ambitions.

5.4.3 Concluding remarks

Whilst Nordenfelt acknowledges the support, influences and restraints put on the individual by the social, cultural and natural environment, he argues for an understanding of humans as primarily individual agents, which he holds to set their norms and values of action according to their own, self-determined goals.

The notion of the individual as an always personal *and* organic construct, a notion signalling a more complex integrative analysis of personhood, is not present in his discourse (nor is it present in any of the previous accounts of health). Nordenfelt acknowledges that as gendered, bodily agents humans might pursue natural goals such as survival and reproduction; but against Boorse, he says if they do so, then not due to their being natural and determined by nature, but due to their own autonomous choice over their bodies.

Nordenfelt's account of health places him in a wider political tradition which understands the human being first as a self-normative individual though contextualised in a network of social relations. Instead, where one views the self as *intrinsically* in relation and interaction with social, cultural and natural factors, and where one acknowledges *the integration* of these different dimensions in the life of the human being, one is unable simply to conceive of the self's goals of happiness as the result of his or her self's autonomous choices. These and similar were explored with St Augustine in the previous chapter.

Clearly, the advantage of Nordenfelt's interpretation is to allow medical practice and health care more generally to centre on the personal needs, desires, views and interpretative accounts of the patient, which are behind the initial choice of actively seeking the clinical encounter. The doctor in turn is seen not as the paternalist authority that administers treatment (or indeed offers repair) but as the enabler: where possible, he or she enables the patient's life goal achievements.

However, the question remains whether a common (social, cultural, political or indeed natural) underpinning of health (and of medicine) can be recognised in such subjective interpretations, or whether clinicians are expected to react to individual demands only. And how could medicine practically be organised to help humans to fulfil their many individual goals? And what does this mean for the shared body of medical knowledge, to which Boorse contributed, and for medical morality, the shared moral code of conduct for the medical profession as enshrined in the *Hippocratic Oath* or the *Declaration of Helsinki*?

---

737 Mordacci, "Health as an Analogical Concept", 481.

Robert Mordacci remarks that Nordenfelt's account opens "the way to a certain arbitrariness."[738] As a consequence, it cannot be foundational for a common body of knowledge and an understanding of generally recognised professional duties or of the moral nature of society's scientific activity *en large*, Mordacci argues. Can medical practice work as an entirely individualised enterprise? Some common reference points and generally accepted goals seem important not only as basis for a common code for professional ethics (medical morality) but moreover as a basis of nationally shared health care systems.

---

738 Mordacci, "Health as Analogical Concept", 483.

6. CONCLUSIONS FOR CONTEMPORARY MEDICINE

Against the background of the practical shortcomings of the philosophical accounts of health, which stem from their fragmentary anthropological foundation, the chapter before us sets out to recover an understanding of health and medical healing which integrates the complexities of the natural-bodily, personal-social and moral-spiritual dimensions of human ontology, hence, allows medicine to account for the patient as a personal and bodily being. It will do so by engaging with contemporary Christian writers and by going over the previous dialogues with writers past and present.

Exegetical analysis of early Christian texts developed how Christian writers of the first millennium reflected on the relationship between theological and rational claims to truth and knowledge, and how their views ranged from the more negative scepticism of Tatian to the positive taking up and transforming of medicine by the Cappadocian Fathers. All writers valued spiritual health and healing as humanity's union with God and the ultimate end of human living and dying. The foregoing exegesis drew out how the health of the body is a good subordinate to the goods of the soul and relative to the absolute goodness of its giver. It elicited how in their striving for health, happiness and joy human beings are orientated towards the fullness of life promised in the future redemption.

Yet this study does neither seek to approach the topic of health from within one particular Christian tradition nor does it present one Christian tradition comprehensively. Whilst it draws extensively on an Augustinian anthropology, it is also open to Orthodox theology and the Eastern Church Fathers. Also, in drawing on the writings of theology's philosophical predecessors in the area of health and medicine (Galen of Pergamon in particular) as well as taking on contemporary philosophical and theological health debates it does not look at Christian theology in isolation from its ancestry or present day companions.

Comparing and contrasting interpretations of health that influenced medicine in its very beginnings on the one hand and help to analyse its present state on the other, allows us to identify gaps, which are addressed with Augustine as well as more contemporary theologians such as Karl Barth, Stanley Hauerwas, and H. Tristram Engelhardt in his recent guise as an Orthodox bioethicist.

In the end, I offer conclusions as to what it means *to be healthy* (rather than to *have health*) and how to *understand* health. These conclusions draw on the analysis offered in chapters three to five, and take up some of the ideas pointed out while engaging with contemporary theological reflections on health. They will be read against the use made of the concept of health in the UK documents on human embryonic stem cell research, in particular the notion of health as bodily repair, and the view of health's value as trumping the value of early human life.

I will elicit the practical importance of the body-soul union as set out by Augustine for a fully connected understanding medicine has of the patient's health, both in research and in the clinical encounter. If oriented towards the patient's life in the body-soul union, the pursuit of health is a good even if it comes at the (temporary) expense of other goods and joys of life. Yet where particular practices of medical research and/or clinical treatment convey an understanding of health and healing that fails to acknowledge the nature of the body as integrating personal particularities, these practices cease to be oriented towards the good of bodily health to which the exegesis of Augustine's anthropology gives rise.

6.1 CONTEMPORARY CHRISTIAN VOICES ON HEALTH AND HEALING

The following will see us engage with Karl Barth's views on abundant human life, health, medicine, and the relationship of the individual to God and fellow humans, H. Tristram Engelhardt as Orthodox Christian bioethicist on issues of bodily and spiritual health and the Orthodox tradition of spiritual healing as well as Stanley Hauerwas on the importance of the church for medical practice as a community able to sustain the presence the sick. In conversing with these figures, I seek to bring out how the positions presented above are in line with as well as differ – at times prominently – from the interpretations and views offered by our contemporaries. Against this background I will move on to develop an approximation of how health might be understood in the contemporary context of medical practice and morality when approached from a perspective that seeks to take seriously God's word in Scripture and the Christian tradition.

6.1.1 Health and the individual-social dimension of life: Karl Barth

When Michael Banner opens his rendering of Christian anthropology with a view to moral issues at the beginning and end of life with the New Testament text, "Fear not; for I am the first, and the last, and the living one"[739] what he emphasises is that we need not fear where we assent to the "word of liberation and judgement"[740] that comes with the reality of Jesus Christ as man and God incarnate. Christ transcends the *temporal* limits of natural, created history. In him past, present and future are one. But, as Banner points out, this affirmation of Christ as the lord of time does not come as an esoteric reflection. Instead, it is made in connection with the great 'fear not' – "the word spoken at the becoming flesh of the 'I am', to shepherds, to Mary and to Joseph."[741] What the Gospel text says, then, is

---

739 Revelation 1:17; Banner, *Christian Ethics and Contemporary Moral Problems*, 48 ff.
740 Ibid., 51.
741 Ibid., 50.

that in Christ's *time-transcending presence* is revealed "the mystery that [...] God intends to be gracious to his creation"[742] at all times.

A second New Testament passage central to Christian anthropology and moral thought reads, "I came that they may have life and have it abundantly."[743] Here, Jesus Christ, the time-transcendent, proclaims and affirms both the gift of life, temporal and finite as well as its fullness in the eschatological future. Such fullness means the redemption of human history, the overcoming of suffering and pain, the fulfilment of human desiring. In Jesus' proclamation of abundance, the gift of life is posited over death, the joy of life over the fear of death, and health over disease. As we have seen, this proclamation of *abundance of life* (also: fullness or completeness) figured prominently in the early Church writers. Fathers as different as Tatian, Tertullian, Basil, and Augustine all emphasised 'health of the soul' or 'spiritual healing' which rests in union with God as humanity's highest good.

Tatian focused on the vertical dimension of human life, the relationship of the body to the soul to the spirit to God: only where the supernatural in humans is oriented (and subordinated) to the divine Creator *true* human (as opposed to mere animal) life is possible. Whilst accepting the reality of the body, Tertullian saw medicine as a secondary mode of healing and underlined the primary importance of spiritual health and healing through the sacraments, which alone can lead to complete well-being. Basil, who firmly placed medicine within God's order of salvation and recommended it to all Christians, strongly underlined that the physician himself was no saviour, and that only through faith in God will humans be lead to the complete happiness in the *eschaton*. For Augustine, knowledge of God's love situated inwardly in the soul needed to come prior to the knowledge of natural processes: only the continuous revelation of this love in past, present, and future and the soul's movement towards it, as well as its renewal and regeneration through it, will lead to everlasting (hence, real) happiness, fearlessness, joy, and well-being.

Abundance and fullness of life, Christ's time-transcending promise to humanity, is the end for which humanity instinctively yearns and towards it acts. From this promise, present life receives its direction, shape, and order. It is from a perspective of completeness given to humans in Christ that states of life such as health and disease, joy and suffering need to be explored.

This perspective of completeness and abundance is, too, what twentieth century Protestant theologian Karl Barth had in mind as he approached medicine's end of health from a theological perspective, that is, from the perspective of *human completeness in Christ*. Such anthropology Karl Barth carries out in section 55 of the *Church Dogmatics* where he introduces human life *in Christ* as the real, concrete, and complete perspective from which the meaning of human health and medical healing can be understood.

---

742 Banner, *Christian Ethics and Contemporary Moral Problems*, 50.
743 John 10:10.

Health thus understood is the invitation to be truly human: it enables us to be

> "Man and not animal or plant, man not wood or stone, man and not a thing or the exponent of
> an idea, man in the satisfaction of his instinctive needs, man in the use of his reason, in
> loyalty to his individuality, in the knowledge of its limitations, man in his determination for
> work and knowledge, and above all in his relation to God and his fellow-men in the proffered
> act of freedom."[744]

The psycho-physical dimension of sickness and health for Barth is only secondary
and subordinated to the primary or ethical dimension, in which consists true human-ness.

> "A man can of course orientate himself seriously, but only secondarily, on this or that psychi-
> cal or physical element of health in contrast to sickness. But *primarily* he will always orien-
> tate himself in this contrast on his own being as man, on his assertion, preservation and re-
> newal (and all this in the form of activity) *as a subject*. In all his particular decisions and
> measures, if they are to be meaningful, he must have a primary concern to confirm his power
> to be as man and to deny the lack of power to be this."[745]

It is striking, perhaps especially in the context of modern scientific medicine, that
Barth's account of health in section 55 of the *Church Dogmatics*, a section entitled 'Freedom for Life', does not begin with a descriptive definition of health in
terms of its physical or psychical reference points such as body, mind, or soul.
Instead, Barth focuses on health's purpose: health serves our individual existence
– the latter being more than the sum total of psycho-physical functioning. In
understanding health as serving human life, Barth moves human life to the centre
of his reflection on health. And in situating health in the context of grace, he
understands life as it corresponds to, and is established by, God in Christ as the
reality upon which the meaning of health is founded.

The distinct perspective from which to approach health and medicine, then, is
anthropological – what does it mean to be human? – what does it mean to live a
truly human life? For Karl Barth the answer lies "in response to God", which includes "reflection of God" as John Paul II puts it. Humans can only "reflect" God
in the *created unity of body and soul*. For both Barth and John Paul II, a human
person is not just a spiritual being.

> "A human being has a body. Therefore the interior acts of knowing and willing, powers of a
> person's soul, should find expression in and through the body. Further, a human person's
> consciousness will mirror or reflect everything he does within himself (interior conscious acts:
> willing and knowing) and the expression of his interior acts through the body."[746]

Whilst the ability to express love in and through the body has been severely impaired through sin, the union of body *and* soul has not been lost. The body is at all
times subjective and personal. In humans, John Paul II says in the *Theology of the
body*, it is never "just a question of the body (intended as an organism, in the somatic sense) but of man, who expresses himself through that body and in this

---

744 Barth, *Church Dogmatics* III/4, 357 (my italics).
745 Ibid., 359.
746 Hogan/LeVoir, *Covenant of Love,* 40.

sense is, I would say, that body."[747] Humans express themselves in and through bodies. They are *personalised* bodies who pursue ends beyond survival and repro-duction. And in a world after the Fall, where the body-soul union is often experi-enced as broken, the restoration of health belongs to the broader narrative of sal-vation: as the New Testament healings indicate, the apostles' miraculous healing belongs to their ministry of making known salvation through Christ.

Barth pursues this lead when he says that good medical practice is the doc-tor's assistance to overcoming bodily obstacles to full life. The doctor's resistance to illness follows from her obedience to God's command: she is not capitulating in the face of sickness.

> "To capitulate before it, to allow it to take its course, can never be obedience but only dis-obedience towards God. In harmony with the will of God what man ought to will in face of this whole realm of the left hand and therefore in face of sickness can only be final resist-ance."[748]

Barth sees the doctor's responsibility to the patient as part of humanity's overall responsibility before God. Hers is a responsibility based on the distinct academic knowledge of disease causes and ways of treatment. Yet there might be times, Barth stresses, for the doctor to respond to the divine command in a manner that requires disposing of her specific academic knowledge: in awareness of the limits of human reason and in faith, she will know that ultimately she cannot extend the limits of life, cannot eliminate mortality. She might be able at least to make the hardship bearable in order to enable the patient to lead his life as a *human being*. Having done this to the best of her ability, the doctor should withdraw, Barth says.[749] If, with God's help, physical sickness is fought victoriously, the kernel of *real* health might be revealed:

> "This kernel, namely that it is good for man to live a limited and impeded life and to be aware of the fact that, when he has exercised and used his strength and power in obedience, he must return them to the One who has lent them to him."[750]

Following Barth, physicians are asked to fulfil their tasks in the knowledge of the importance and the limitations of their profession.

> He will be a better doctor the more consciously he realises his limitations in this respect. For in this way he can draw the attention of others to the fact that the main thing in getting well is something in which neither he nor any human meas-ure can help. If he is a Christian doctor, in certain cases he will explicitly draw attention to this fact.[751]

Whilst we find aspects of much of the Church Father's writings present in Barth's discussion of health and medical healing – above all the limitedness of

---

747 John Paul II, *Theology of the Body*, 203.
748 Barth, *Church Dogmatics* III/4, 367.
749 Ibid., 362.
750 Ibid., 374.
751 Ibid., 361.

medical power based on the understanding of life as loaned[752] – at least three points seem important to raise in response to his account.

(1) Barth places a strong emphasis on *health as a service to human life* by which he means *the individual human being's life*. Health is a service to my particular life, in that it enables me, when I am in good health, to live as this particular woman in the satisfaction of my instinctive needs, in the use of my reason, in loyalty to my individuality, in the knowledge of its limitations, in my determination for work and knowledge. And since good health stems from my relation to God, it enables me to live in relation to him and my fellow humans, and to fulfil my human-ness in this relation.[753] Whilst it is clear, therefore, that the healthy human life lived in Christ at all times *includes* the relation to one's "fellow-men in the proffered act of freedom,"[754] Barth does not spell out explicitly that health as enabling true human-ness finds its most pertinent expression precisely *in one's relationship with one's fellow humans*.

(2) Yet this is what Augustine seems to have had in mind where he talks about the soul as the image of God's love (a relational love, which connects God with the self and the others) and about health of the soul as the process of restoration of this image, which enables a life lived in love of God, self, and the other.

Health, Augustine's hierarchical view of health suggests, is not primarily the orientation of humans as subjects (as Barth says above) but the expression of human-ness in their relationship with others. Such interpretation of health allows Augustine to recommend human acts oriented towards the other as acts leading to happiness – without making our possibility for such acts *dependent on our bodily state*.

Whilst Barth is right to stress that bodily health serves me in that it makes it easier to be there for others (would I want to prepare breakfast for my daughter when ill with flu?), Augustine excels Barth (and follows Paul) where he underlines that paradoxically though it seems it is especially where I am bodily weak that *I am sustained by God's grace*. As the above examples showed, Augustine was acutely aware that illness and above all pain often bring with it the tendency to withdraw onto one's self and to show concern for one's body alone. Precisely in facing this temptation of love of self he emphasised the unimaginably greater power of God's love which can free us to encountering the other.

(3) With Augustine's relational understanding of the soul in process of renewal – starting with the moment of baptism and from then onwards determining one's life with intermitting periods of ill-health and health, or greater and lesser realisation of God's love – comes an emphasis on love and philanthropic actions. *Philanthropeia* was, too, the hinge around which turned Basil's actions against disease and social exclusion.

Yet such explicit emphasis on philanthropy (or cure *and* care) is alien to Barth's treatment of the subject. For Barth, medicine is to be approved and de-

752 Ibid., 374.
753 Barth, *Church Dogmatics* III/4, 357 (my italics).
754 Ibid.

fended for it shows *obedience to God's command to life*: a doctor's (and patient's) resistance to sickness, which belongs to the realm of the left hand,[755] is in accordance with God's command.

Whilst the outcome might be not too different (that is, in both instances medicine is recommended as a practice in accordance with God's will), it does appear to be a marked difference whether we focus on Christ's curing and caring for others as the model for full human existence (as does Basil, and against the background of his view of the soul, also Augustine) or on the fulfilling of the divine command pronounced to the individual to live his or her life in true human-ness (which only in a second step includes acts of charity towards the other).

In the first instance, the emphasis is first and foremost on Christ's actions towards the other – here and now as proleptic of the future salvation of humanity; in the second instance, focus is on God's promise of life to the individual, a life which will always be incomplete in the here and now, and fulfilled in eschaton. Such a life will include the presence to the other, yet such presence is not as intimately linked with a fulfilled human existence as it is in the first instance.

However, what unites both positions is the understanding of human life as incomplete and unfulfilled at present; as moving towards abundance in Christ; as living under the promise of salvation. The following section will look at health and medicine from this perspective of salvation through engaging with recent work by H. Tristram Engelhardt, now writing as a convert to Orthodox Christianity.

6.1.2 Health and medicine in pursuit of salvation: Orthodox theology

As an Orthodox Catholic or "traditional Christian"[756] united in belief and worship with "the Patriarch of Antioch, the Archbishop of Athens and of all Greece, the Patriarch of Moscow, the Catholicos of Georgia, the Pope of Alexandria and all Africa, and the Metropolitan of Washington, not to mention the bishop of Dallas and the South, among others"[757] H. Tristram Engelhardt would readily agree with Barth at least in one crucial respect: that health is an important good, and that to avoid suffering and to postpone death is generally good, too. However, he emphasises, "It is not worldly cure, care, and health that are most important. They

---

755 Barth, *Church Dogmatics* III/4, 367.
756 Engelhardt, *Foundations of Christian Bioethics*, xvii. Engelhardt admits to using the term 'traditional Christianity' as a code word for Orthodox Christianity and Christian reflections articulated in the first millennium. The term invites today's audiences, Engelhardt says, to enter into the religious experience alive in texts, prayers, moral and spiritual concerns of the first thousand years. Engelhardt perceives traditional Christianity as the root of Western theology and philosophy yet as fundamentally out of step with the Christian religions of the West in that it is liturgical and ascetic. Traditional Christianity celebrates the gift of the Scriptures as of reason inspired by faith but does not recognise them as essential to Christianity.
757 Engelhardt, *Foundations of Christian Bioethics*, xvi.

have enduring significance only if they lead to the only true cure of death: salvation."[758]

Whilst rejecting mainline Protestantism as well as forms of Roman Catholicism for accommodating the pretensions of secular culture and fostering the values and concerns of secularism, Engelhardt applauds Barth for not founding moral theology on natural law principles and rational accounts of morality.[759]

Like Barth, he looks to the foundations of Christianity in developing his account of ethics, yet unlike Barth, he does not set the word in Scripture and reasoning developed from it at the centre of faith but draws on the Church writers of the first millennium, "traditional Christianity". Traditional Christianity "is grounded in unbroken veridical *experience* of God."[760] For Engelhardt, *experience* of God, as opposed to reasoning about God is at the heart of Orthodox theology. Orthodoxy is not primarily a theology

> "Of academicians advancing their considered intuitions. It is a theology won by asceticism and through experience of the God Who unites His theologians over space and across the millennia. It understands that to know truly is not a matter of discursive or scholastic reasoning, but of changing the knower and of being granted illumination by God."[761]

Only this traditional Christianity, that is, Christianity drawing on the texts of the early Church and the Church Fathers of the East[762] can be the foundation of Christian bioethics or medical ethics as a lived ethic.[763] Where it speaks to medicine and health care, only traditional Christianity with its orientation towards the kingdom of God relocates all medical concerns with reference to the struggle to holiness,[764] thus is able to re-orient, indeed to transform, secular medicine's practices and actions – without being transformed by these practices in return. This problem Engelhardt encounters in most other Christian moral approaches to secular medicine.

> "If reason is at the centre of theology, one will rationally reconstruct the content of any Christian bioethics in the image and likeness of secular moral rationality. [...] If Scripture is at the core of theology, its authoritative claims will be deconstructed through text-critical and sociohistorical reassessments of the Scriptures, thus rendering it congenial to the assumptions of our age."[765]

---

758 Engelhardt, *Foundations of Christian Bioethics,* 354.
759 Ibid., 57 (footnote 61).
760 Ibid., xvi.
761 Ibid.
762 Engelhardt distinguishes between the West and the East, the former for him characterised as seeking understanding mostly through discursive reflection, not noetic knowledge. He perceives many historical roots of this difference, one of which being the influence of Augustine, "whose understanding of doctrine and whose aspirations to intellectual knowledge were not the same as those of the Church that produced the Councils" (ibid., 202).
763 Ibid., xvi.
764 Ibid., 237.
765 Ibid., xvi. Whilst the first is launched against Roman Catholic bioethics, the latter attacks forms of contemporary Protestantism; both concerns, present thought they are in mainline Catholicism and Protestantism and not without contingency either, are not necessarily the case as the examples in this section show.

Traditional Christian bioethics which Engelhardt proposes takes its character and content from a life directed to union with God, to becoming God-like. Christian bioethics is not a set of rules. It is integral to a liturgical life leading to union with a fully transcendent God – in this sense it always is a liturgically and experientially "lived ethics".[766] Indeed, such emphasis on the union with God and liturgical practice accords completely with the ideas drawn from the writings of the Cappadocian Fathers.

Engelhardt translates their writings on the orientation of life in the contemporary context when he speaks out against medicine as an idol – which, for him, is what medicine is in danger of becoming where its practices take place outside of the traditional Christian understanding of life, that is, without orientation toward God. "Without this orientation, which must aim at God through the crucifixion and resurrection, medicine's place in culture threatens to be dangerously distorted."[767]

For Engelhardt, medical centres and hospitals have become a focus of economic investment and energy in contemporary Western societies; they have taken on "the cultural roles that cathedrals once claimed in the West."[768] Whereas in the Middle Ages, people would have been keen to sell all their possession for the building of a cathedral, altar, church window etc. in the hope of securing eternal salvation for themselves or their families, many will now sell all they have to secure a few more years of life promised by medical advances.

> "Medicine possesses a commanding place in contemporary culture. Medical centres are now the place where many, if not most, seek to resolve the problems of their sexuality, suffering, dying, and death."[769]

The monumental projects of the Middle Ages and the present times disclose what a society takes to be important life goals: the transcending creator, or the immanent creature. Where medieval cathedrals or temples were built to glorify the greatness of a transcendent God, hospitals are built for the restoration and preservation of immanent life through natural knowledge, therefore have no orientation beyond the medical understanding of life, health, and well-being that is on offer.

In his critique of an increasing medicalisation of society, as well as in the imagery used, Engelhardt clearly does not occupy a solitary position: as mentioned earlier, it has philosophical predecessors in the 1960s and 1970s (Michael Foucault and Ivan Illich being prominent at the time) but also in today's culture. Manfred Lütz,[770] a contemporary Roman Catholic psychiatrist and psychoanalyst, speaks of hospitals as the cathedral of the twentieth century[771] or the inner temple of the new "health religion" as he terms it not without irony.[772]

---

766 Engelhardt, *Foundations of Christian Bioethics,* 236.
767 Ibid., 316.
768 Ibid., 317.
769 Ibid.
770 M. Lütz, *Lebenslust* (München 2002).
771 Ibid., 56.
772 Ibid., 57.

Where the full meaning of life is beyond death, medicine cannot be the art most needed for a healthy life; it has a role to play, and Christians may engage in medical interventions, yet one's focus should first rest on 'spiritual health', and on interventions that foster the spiritual life and journey toward union with God. With reference to Basil the Great's views on medicine and healing, Engelhardt underlines as appropriate focus the way to holiness, to becoming God-like, not the saving or preserving of life. Where health care practices distract humans from the proper end of union with God they should be avoided. Nevertheless, Engelhardt emphasises in much the same way as Basil that health care remains important – as a temporary expedient, and in dedication to God and others. "To be philanthropic was to be God-like".[773] It is from this perspective that Engelhardt re-examines how health care professionals should relate to their patients with spiritual integrity. He addresses topics such as withholding or withdrawing treatment, informed consent, allocation of resources, transplantation, euthanasia, yet also issues of reproductive technologies, including cloning and the use of embryos in research.

Whilst Engelhardt underlines human life's orientation towards holiness, hence, the spiritual dimension of human life without spelling out an Orthodox Christian anthropology, Stanley S. Harakas, a prominent Orthodox theologian and ethicist, underlines that Eastern Orthodox Christianity sees body and soul (bodily health and spiritual health) as united and intimately related.[774]

> "To be a human being, then, means to be a fully psychosomatic created being conceived of human parents, endowed with the image of God, and called to realise the potential of the likeness of God in communion with him and with other human beings."[775]

Harakas speaks about the Christian Orthodox attitude to health and medicine against the background of the body-soul union and its being in the image and likeness of God.[776] As regards the mainline Orthodox approach to sickness, health, and medicine, Harakas underlines that physical, emotional, and spiritual (or moral) disturbances are considered holistically. They are all within the purview of the physician. Equally, body and spirit are both concerns for the church. Spiritual and liturgical efforts at healing are encouraged at all times. The Orthodox church sees the healing power of God and the ministrations of physicians and rational medicine in essential harmony. This being the case, it has recourse to spiritual means of healing such as prayer, sacraments (above all the sacrament of holy unction which is dedicated to healing exclusively) as well as the appeal to saints while accepting and embracing at the same time rational forms of medical knowledge.

In this context, Harakas directs attention to the Byzantine tradition of clergy-physicians, where spiritual and rational healing were brought together in one person. He emphasises that even today there are various examples of ordained physicians.[777] Further, he explains the importance of healing through saints (most

---

773 Harakas, *Health in the Orthodox Tradition*, 64.
774 Ibid., 28.
775 Ibid., 62.
776 Ibid., 60–63.
777 Ibid., 80.

prominently Cosmas and Damian, patron saints of doctors[778]) in Orthodox Christianity. Their ways of healing (touch, prayer, dust and so on) were in accordance with the healings accounted for in the New Testament (*vide supra*).[779] Often shrines were constructed in the honour of saints and where found in monasteries where hospitals were also established.

> "In most cases, neither the monks nor the physicians nor the patients and their families perceived a sharp line of demarcation between the shrine and the hospital, between what we are calling here spiritual healing and rational medicine."[780]

Harakas underlines that also today nearly all liturgical services of the Orthodox Church (in particular the sacraments of baptism and Eucharist) include some mention of physical healing.[781]

It is impossible at this stage to give an in-depth account of spiritual healing in the Orthodox tradition and contemporary Orthodox Christianity. This is also not an exploration of these issues as regards theological presuppositions and underlying doctrines of human-ness, holiness, and salvation. Yet the prevailing emphasis on spiritual healing is, perhaps, the biggest difference between not only today's Orthodox Christianity and contemporary Protestantism, but also between the Church Fathers and academic Protestantism, at least as it is taught in the Western context. The Orthodox Christian tradition appears to embrace readily healing dimensions such as exorcisms, healings of the saints, sacramental healing and rational medicine, and understands them as dimensions of human existence within the saving, redeeming, and sanctifying work of Christ.

Mainline Protestantism in its academic variant on the other hand, despite its rootedness in the word of Scripture as opposed to rational arguments, natural laws or the Roman Catholic ecclesial tradition, appears at a loss when it comes to responding for instance to the exorcisms and Gospel healings. Whilst it is able to respond positively to rational medicine on grounds of the goodness of the body, what to make of the call for spiritual healings so prominent in the Church Fathers as well as Orthodox Christianity remains an open question, clearly in need of further investigation.

---

778 The twins Cosmas and Damian protected the fields and helped the infirm. Their bones were often believed to be resting places of the Holy Spirit, and dust from their graves was a valuable relic to ward off or cure sickness. At the time of the Byzantine Empire, Cosmas and Damian were worshipped by both Eastern and Western Christianity. "We find their names at the end of the Communicantes of the Roman Mass; they have a place together with the martyrs." (Skrobucha, *Patrons of the doctors*, 9). Churches and chapels were dedicated to them in the fifth century, pilgrimages organised to their graves. "The brothers appeared in person, or cured at least the patients in the hospital connected with their church in Constantinople. Sometimes they also made known their message of healing to friends or neighbours of the diseased. Oftentimes the brothers were recognised by the sick who knew them from icons and Cosmas and Damian also performed healings by means of icons. One woman who had the icon of the Saints on the walls of her home once was taken ill when alone. She scratched some of the colour from the icons and added some to a drink and became well" (ibid., 17–18).
779 Harakas, *Health in the Orthodox Tradition*, 84.
780 Ibid., 85.
781 Ibid., 90.

However, one aspect of healing central to Orthodox Christianity's healing dimensions, namely the liturgical presence of the church, has been explored more recently by contemporary Methodist theologian Stanley Hauerwas in his article "Salvation and Health: Why Medicine Needs the Church". Before moving onto an analysis of Hauerwas' article, I will start by reflecting with Albert Camus in *The Plague* and Dietrich Bonhoeffer in his *Ethics* on the relationship between theology and medicine more generally.

6.1.3 Relationship of theology and medicine: Stanley Hauerwas

In the immediate contact with human suffering, doctor Rieux in Camus' *Plague* describes himself as working side by side with the priest towards the *relief* of suffering, and that is towards *health*. Yet in his medical function, the doctor sees himself as primarily concerned with the body's *temporal* health whereas Father Paneloux in his priestly function understands himself as primarily concerned with the soul's *eternal* health.

Unlike some of the Orthodox Christian physicians, the "clergyphysicians" which Stanley Harakas had in mind above, Father Paneloux and doctor Rieux both assume a duality of functions: medicine refers to the sphere of the body, the natural, the world; theology refers to the soul, the supernatural, the divine. For doctor Rieux and Father Paneloux, there is not *one* ordered and oriented reality embracing body and soul but a dual reality: there is the reality of the body which comprises the body's own kinds of diseases and which is strictly demarcated from the reality of the soul with its own kind of diseases, health and death.

Of course, this view of two distinct realities begs the difficult question as to their relationship: how does the body relate to the soul, the sphere of the natural to the supernatural, and the clinic to the church? Does each require its own epistemology, its own semantics, and its own discourse? Do we indeed approach the supernatural through the word of God in Holy Scripture or canonised scriptural interpretation[782] alone whilst we approach the natural through the canon of western medicine as available in medical handbooks[783] or through the knowledge of the natural sciences more generally? The separation of reality into the psychophysical and spiritual, the natural and supernatural, the sacred and profane tends to a compartmentalised kind of understanding and acting.

Dietrich Bonhoeffer pointed out in his *Ethics* that to conceive of reality as two distinct spheres means, ultimately, humans live either a spiritual life without participation in the world or a worldly life without spiritual reference. A dual view of reality creates a world which claims its own laws against the spiritual. It creates a church which is unable to set her morality and agency in relation to the surrounding society. Such a church is unable to call for a Christian life in the world.[784] It is

---

782 Cf. Camus, *The Plague*, 78.
783 Ibid., 36; 44.
784 Bonhoeffer, *Ethik*, 209.

unable to address the State, to engage with politics, to confront economic and social injustice, to talk to the medicine and biotechnological practices. Nor can the goods these institutions have to offer address the church. And this is the social crisis in which doctor Rieux and Father Paneloux specifically find themselves in Camus' *Plague*.

From the day at the boy's deathbed, Paneloux begins work on a short essay entitled *Is a Priest Justified in Consulting a Doctor?* Following this work, he proclaims in his next sermon a faith that presents humans with the polarised choice of *either* the world *or* God, either nature or spirit, either medicine or theology. We need to – God being the author of the plague – "choose either to hate God or to love God"[785] Paneloux says. We can either seek eternal redemption or the natural, temporal goods of the world such as bodily health. Either we withdraw from the world, which is utterly fallen, thereby seeking salvation, or we live a material life in the material world until death puts an end to it.

Such faith echoes an approach to Christian faith epitomised by the existentialism of Kierkegaard. It assumes for theology its own logic and reason, implacably opposed to human, fallen, logic and reason. It is not the faith presented by the writers of the first millennium or indeed their present day followers. Yet Paneloux stresses, that it is "*illogical* for a priest to call in a doctor."[786] For him, faith is a faith in the face of the absurd, that is, in the face of suffering, which according to *human* reason must entail the loss of faith in a loving God according to the possibilities of traditional non-eschatological theodicy. When seeing somebody's life destroyed by illness we face the decision of believing *totally* or of denying everything.[787] Either we believe in the absoluteness of God's love and goodness *despite appearances* or we deny God's omnipotence, the goodness of his creation and of human existence therein. We face an *either-or-decision*.

To believe God's love *and* accept a doctor's intervention, on the other hand, springs from a faith that acknowledges the contingency of life, the full, eschatological redemption of history, and relies on both ecclesial and non-ecclesial modes of practice. For Paneloux though, such a faith can be but a fallen compromise. A faith that allows for both the natural and the supernatural modes of action is unable to believe *totally,* to decide *ultimately.* There is no middle course, Paneloux says. The choice is *either* Christ *or* the world. It is either Christ *without the world*, or the world *without Christ*.[788] Where we decide in the face of suffering to believe in Christ and the *absoluteness* of God's love we *absolutely* renounce the world. Accordingly, we have to reject all medical assistance that might have saved our eyes or preserved our life. Christ alone bears salvation, a salvation borne through the church. The faith Father Paneloux presents us with is not a faith in Christ as God *in* the world. Therefore it is not a faith in *Christ with the world*.

---

785 Camus, *The Plague*, 186.
786 Ibid., 187 (my italics).
787 Ibid.
788 Bonhoeffer, *Ethics*, 58.

As has been shown above such polarisation was alien to the vast majority of early Church writers as well as contemporary Orthodox theology with its tradition of clergy-physicians. Yet we find ourselves presented with such polarising tendency, the choice between biased, subjective theology *or* objective, neutral, factual natural sciences, in much public debate on modern scientific and medical achievements. In being *a choice* it fits itself smoothly into the current concerns of Western capitalist-pluralist societies lacking moral consensus and emphasising the individual's right to choice. It leads us to believe that societal peace lies in the state's protection of our right to lifestyle choices, here in an existential context. The domains of medicine and the church, analogous to state and church, must be kept apart in order to safeguard the smooth-running efficiency of Western societies; medicine must fit consumer demands (and vice-versa), not some metaphysical soft talk about love.

Yet Stanley Hauerwas turns the view of *either-or-choice* on its head. For him, the question is not whether a priest could be justified in consulting a doctor (as has been the question for Christian writers of the first millennium including Augustine) or whether priests' and doctors' work is in essential harmony (the idea of a union of both in the clergyphysician as explored by Harakas being the prime example). Hauerwas perceives of medicine and the church as meeting in their concern with the sufferer: they both seek to be present to the one in pain. And here, Hauerwas argues, it is logical for the *doctor* to call in the church, since the church as a community with habits of *fearless presence to the sufferer* is able to sustain the doctor's all too often isolated and isolating presence at the hospital bed.

This thesis, then, is original in that it is able to argue for the presence of the church *without diminishing the good of medicine and bodily healing*, which is one of the risks intrinsic to any hierarchical view of health as developed by the early Church and above all Augustine. At the same time, in taking the church community as starting point, he does not diminish the primary role of Christianity in healing, which is the risk inherent to any modern variation of Christianity that seeks to follow the argumentative structure of rational sciences.

In full, the title of Hauerwas's 1985 article to which I refer here reads, "Salvation and health: Why medicine needs the church." It is published in a volume edited by E.E. Shelp on the relationship of theology and the (at least by theological standards) young discipline of bioethics. The volume is part of the series *Philosophy and Medicine*. The article brings out core themes that Hauerwas develops further in the 1993 monograph *Naming the Silences: God, Medicine and the Problem of Suffering*. On both occasions, Hauerwas attempts to understand the nature and kinds of suffering, the role and nature of medicine in human lives, and human understanding of God.

In accordance with the contention of the significance of the narrative for rational ethical reflection,[789] which is original for Hauerwas' work, he starts by of-

---

789 Cf. Hauerwas/Burrell, "From System to Story: An Alternative Pattern for Rationality in Ethics", in: Engelhardt/Callahan: *The Roots of Ethics. Science, Religion and Values* (1981), 75–105. See also *Naming the Silences* where "much of this book is made up of stories about

fering a text and a story. The text is from Scripture, Job 2:11–13, and recounts Job's friends coming together to condole with Job and comfort him in his suffering and loss. "And they sat with him on the ground for seven days and seven nights, and no one spoke a word to him, for they saw that his suffering was very great."[790] To start with a metaphysical source is, Hauerwas remarks, rare for those "who turn their attention to issues of medicine"[791] which is, it is claimed, a discipline based on the principles and rules of nature. Hauerwas leaves the passage from Job and its wider importance for medical morality and the relation of theology and medicine uncommented to start with, and instead continues by telling the story of one of his earliest friends.

Bob phoned one Sunday morning to tell Hauerwas that he had found his mother dead. She had committed suicide. Despite feeling awkward and not knowing what to say or do, Hauerwas went to see his friend. All he could do was to be present much as Job's friends where present to him in his suffering. "For the rest of that day and that night we stayed together. I do not remember what we said, but I do remember that it was inconsequential."[792] Yet a few months later the two friends grew apart: "What was standing between us was that day and night we spent together under the burden of a profound sadness."[793]

Both the passage from Job and the story of Bob, the sharing of grief and the experience of separation through grief, are a way into his thesis that "something very much like a church" is needed to sustain medicine's presence to those in pain day in and day out.[794]

It is with this thesis that I am concerned in the following. It takes us back to, and answers questions as to the reality of nature and the nature of medicine, as well as the relation of theology and medicine, and how, from a contemporary Protestant perspective, the presence of the church as a community of care might be essential for medicine's continuous presence at the hospital bed.

For the most of human history medicine and religion were not distinguished, Hauerwas points out with reference to Darrell Amundsen and Gary Ferngren, and their analysis of the Hebrew Bible and the New Testament in "Medicine and Religion: Pre-Christian Antiquity."[795] Based on Amundsen/Ferngren's exploration of Scripture it is not possible, Hauerwas says, "to separate and/or distinguish religion from medicine, on the basis of a distinction between soul and body"[796] for both

---

ill and dying children" (xii) and where the stories are never mere illustrations (2) but its basic 'argument' (xii). Life stories and the manifestation of God's glory in them can help us to understand God's story (ibid.).

790 Job 2:13.
791 Hauerwas, "Salvation and Health", 205.
792 Ibid., 206. On the idea of sharing presence in suffering also Hauerwas, *Naming the Silences*, 151.
793 Hauerwas, "Salvation and Health", 207.
794 Ibid.
795 Cf. Adolf von Harnack's thesis of Christianity as a 'medical religion' – chapter three.
796 Hauerwas, "Salvation and Health", 209.

disciplines know, he claims, "of the inseparability of soul and body."[797] Yet since both disciplines are concerned with the same subject (namely humans in the union of body and soul) "structurally the possibility of conflict between the church and medicine cannot be excluded."[798] Two answers have been suggested to this conflict, both "quite different and equally unsatisfactory,"[799] and he goes on to explore the two alternatives.

"The first underwrites a strong division of labour between medicine and religion by limiting the scope of medicine to the mechanism of the body."[800] It also assumes a division of expertise between the physician and the clergy – here we can recognise Father Paneloux's viewpoint. Where religion is keen to limit medicine to a mechanical understanding and care of the body it itself can shine ethereally as that which is concerned with the soul, the truly good – one of the temptation of Gnosticism and/or Manicheism, as Augustine remarked. Yet such a view eclipses the personal nature of the body on which is grounded the moral nature of medical care; the moral commitment of the physician is *not* to treat physical processes but the particular patient before him or her.

"The other alternative [...] seeks to maintain a close relationship by resacralising medical care"[801] thus, not widening but collapsing the gap between theology and medicine. Indeed, where medicine's ability to cure increases, medicine is tempted to offer a form of salvation of the whole human being. Against this, physicians might rightly maintain that their skills are primarily focussed on the body thus preventing a view that considers medicine as an agency of salvation.[802]

Following on from this, and in contrast to some other theologians writing in medical ethics (for instance, Joseph Fletcher, Paul Ramsey, James Gustafson and James Childress), Hauerwas proposes that moral theologians seeking to secure the moral integrity of medicine need to challenge some of the basic presuppositions of medical practice and care on the basis of their distinctive commitments as theologians.[803] This leaves him to explore the ways in which theologians can go about offering such challenges in dialogue with Alasdair MacIntyre in "Can medicine dispense with a theological perspective on human nature?".

According to MacIntyre, theologians can either decode Christianity in order to make it intelligible to the secularised world (which is precisely what Engelhardt criticised modern Protestantism and Catholicism for) or insist that the secular world must accept Christianity on its own terms (which is what Engelhardt opted for in his "traditional Christian Bioethics" – for him there is no academic discipline 'theology' but only sacred doctrine).

---

797 Hauerwas, "Salvation and Health", 209.
798 Ibid., 210.
799 Ibid.
800 Ibid.
801 Ibid.
802 And it might indeed "be a fundamental judgment on the church's failure to help us locate wherein our salvation lies that so many today seek a salvation through medicine" (Hauerwas, "Salvation and Health", 211).
803 Ibid., 213.

Hauerwas argues with MacIntyre that "to decode turns out to be to destroy"[804] for theologians "inhabit an intellectual universe in which the natural sciences are at home and theology is not."[805]

Yet what is the alternative then for theology in relation to medicine? What about the second option? Here Hauerwas returns to his original text and story "to show how they might offer some solution for helping us to understand how Christian convictions can or should inform the practice of medicine within our current culture"[806] without limiting medicine to the body or resacralising medical care. And immediately it is central for him to clarify that where he talks about religion or theology or Christian convictions, he talks about "the church" that is "a community with cultic practices."[807]

Where we speak about medicine or religion in general terms rather than as specific sets of behaviour and habits embodied by distinct groups of people we distort the character of what we mean to describe, Hauerwas says. For him, the question of the relationship of medicine and theology cannot be posed in abstract terms. What he wants to show is rather why "given the *particular* demands put on those who care for the ill something very much like a church [a *particular* community with ritual practices, A.C.] is necessary to sustain that care."[808]

To develop the point, Hauerwas returns to the phenomenon of pain: "Pain comes in many shapes and sizes and it is never possible to separate the psychological aspects of pain from the organic."[809] Whilst pain always is a very particular experience, and one that cannot be *easily* communicated (as both the example of Job and Hauerwas' friend illustrated), it is entirely *impossible* to experience someone else's pain. Pain is an experience humans share, yet it does not create a shared experience. "What we cannot do is for you to understand and/or experience my pain as mine" so that "our pains isolate us from one another as they create worlds that cut us off from one another."[810] This is one of the burdens of chronic illness, Hauerwas points out. Where it is impossible "to be compassionate year in and year out", people with chronic illnesses (and often their closest relatives and/or friends, too) become alienated of their former friends. Hauerwas concludes, "Exactly because pain is so alienating we are hesitant to admit that we are in pain."[811]

Now, it is to the presence to those in pain that physicians should be fundamentally committed, Hauerwas says. Here, he is not concerned with *why*[812] but

---

804 MacIntyre, "Can Medicine Dispense with Theology", 130.
805 Ibid., 131.
806 Hauerwas, "Salvation and Health", 216.
807 Ibid., 217.
808 Ibid (my italics).
809 Ibid.
810 Ibid., 218.
811 Ibid., 219.
812 Chapters three and four, in particular Basil's account of *philanthropic* care and Augustine's view of *relational* love and commitment to the other, can be taken as explorations of the moral reasons for such commitment in the context of this study.

that they are present to the ones in pain like no other humans, thus forming a bridge between the world of the ill and the healthy.[813] Of course, physicians seek cures; yet every physician also learns the limits of his or her craft and that "the sheer particularity of the patient's illness often defies the best knowledge and skill."[814] Not only is such presence a very difficult task to be carried out day-to-day but also do they deal with an experience which the healthy want to keep at arm's length. "They have seen the world we do not want to see until it is forced on us, and we will accept them into polite community only to the extent they keep that world hidden from us."[815]

Here Hauerwas' argument reaches its crucial stage. For now he faces the question as to how the physician can be present to the ill and the ones in pain "day in day out without learning to dislike them, if not positively detest their smallness in the face of pain."[816] The central question is, then, what *sustains* the presence of medicine in the face of pain and suffering? Empathy would be one possible answer, and Hauerwas views it as necessary though not sufficient. Nor is it sufficient "to account for the acquiring of the skills necessary to sustain that presence in a manner that is not alienating and the source of distrust in a community."[817]

To learn *how* to sustain medicine's presence in the face of suffering and to *determine* both form and content of such presence, humans need *examples* – that is, "a people who have learned to embody such a presence in their lives that it has become the marrow of their habits."[818] And this is precisely what Hauerwas takes the church to be: the community of a people whose habits (ritual and liturgical) include the presence to those in pain. "The church at least claims to be such a community, as it is a group of people called out by a God who we believe is always present to us both in our sin and our faithfulness"[819] – hence, who is present to us both were we are in pain and where we are well. In awareness of God's unfailing presence in the midst of sin and pain, the church community is trained to remember as a communal act their sins and pains. This act can offer a paradigm for "sustaining across time a painful memory so that it acts to heal rather than to divide"[820] as was the case in Job's story and Stanley Hauerwas with his friend Bob. Hauerwas also points to the necessity of prayer: not as a

"Supplement to the insufficiency of our medical knowledge and practice; nor is it some divine insurance policy that our medical skill will work; rather, our prayer is the means that we have to make God present, whether our medical skill is successful or not."[821]

According to Hauerwas, then, the presence of the church which is necessary for medicine's mission of cure and care *is not formal but essential to medicine's*

813 Hauerwas, "Salvation and Health", 220.
814 Ibid.
815 Ibid.
816 Ibid., 221.
817 Ibid.
818 Ibid.
819 Ibid.
820 Ibid., 222.
821 Ibid., 222–223.

caring presence; it also seems to exceed the ritual prayer for those who are sick during mass. What seems at the heart of his thesis is a view of church as a community of people with certain habits – here, the habit of being *fearlessly* present in caring for the one in pain. A community which models its habits on Christ's time-transcending *fear not* ceases to fear the sustained contact with, and exposition to, strangers, socially excluded or sufferers of pain. Its own fearless presence allows it to welcome others who are present to pain, such as medical personnel, and in welcoming lifts the ban of isolation placed on those who are present to pain by the majority of those who fear pain and do not want to be in contact with it. To be welcomed into a community that is able to sustain such presence, will in turn enable physicians to sustain their patient presence at the hospital bed.

Crucial as it seems, a more thorough analysis of Hauerwas' ecclesiology requires more time and space than is possible in the present context. Suffice it to say here that Hauerwas himself references his idea to Augustine, who, after his conversion to Christianity, looked for the conversion of people's hearts, which makes them belong to the community of fellowship between humans and God, a "community of care"[822] for each other. In this community, the church community, Hauerwas concludes, the terror of disease will be absorbed – both for the one who suffers from it, and for the one who is present to him.[823]

6.2 UNDERSTANDING OF HEALTH IN A CONTEMPORARY CONTEXT

Having engaged in the preceding sections with contemporary theologians' contributions to the health debate while drawing out short comings in connection to the theological writings of the first millennium, I now offer summarising conclusions as to what it means *to be healthy* (rather than to *have health*) and as to how to *think about* bodily health (I emphasise *think about* health, for I do not seek to *define* it). These conclusions draw on the analysis offered in chapters three to five, and take up some of the ideas pointed out while engaging with contemporary theological reflections on health. They will be read against the use made of the concept of health in the UK documents on human embryonic stem cell research, in particular the notion of health as bodily repair, and the view of health's value as trumping the value of early human life.

What I develop is an account of health and healing which is largely based on an Augustinian anthropology. I have drawn on the writings of theology's philosophical predecessors in the area of health and medicine (Galen of Pergamon in particular) and have discussed contemporary philosophical and theological health debates (the former in chapter five, the latter in chapters three, four, and six especially). Comparing and contrasting interpretations of health that influenced medicine in its very beginnings on the one hand and helped to analyse its present state

822 Hauerwas, *Naming the Silences*, 53.
823 Ibid.

on the other, allowed me to identify gaps as well as to address them with Augustine and more contemporary theologians.

My claim was that the philosophical accounts of health show how a fragmentary view of human life is bound up with a disconnected view of health – and *vice versa*. In the following, I elicit the practical importance of the body-soul union for a fully connected understanding medicine has of the patient's health, both in research and in the clinical encounter.

Medical research aimed at novel therapies and clinical treatment aimed at health are good actions where they take into account the wider dimensions of human life such as personhood and sociability which are integrated in the body and served by the state of health. If oriented towards the patient's life in the body-soul union, the pursuit of health is a good even if it comes at the (temporary) expense of other goods and joys of life. Yet where particular practices of medical research and/or clinical treatment convey an understanding of health and healing that fails to acknowledge the nature of the body as integrating personal particularities, these practices cease to be oriented towards the good of bodily health to which the exegesis of Augustine's anthropology gives rise.

Bodily health is a *temporal* and *relative* good. It is temporal because life is finite. It is a relative good measured against the good of the soul, which is union with God. Bodily health being relative to the good of the soul, its practical importance (hence, the importance of a particular avenue of research and/or treatment) may be assessed in relation to its service to the good of the soul. In being recognised as a good which serves human life, health may motivate medical action. It may function as research imperative and promote medical action. At the same time its temporal and relative nature limits medical action in that it measures it against the horizon of finitude and divine love.

6.2.1 Health from within the body-soul union

"Health is the strength *to be as man*. It serves human existence in the form of the capacity, vitality and freedom to exercise the psychical and physical functions, just as these themselves are only functions of human existence."[824]

Barth advanced his understanding of health in the late 1950s and early 1960s as part of his overall endeavour to identify human life, action, freedom and community in God's love and freedom. At that time, the notion of human health was not seriously questioned or investigated by neither the medical nor the philosophical profession: as has been shown in chapter three, it was only in the 1970s that the concepts of health and disease became the subject of academic debate in the Anglo-American context.

These philosophical accounts of health did not recognise the individual-personal, cultural, social, and natural dimension of life as *integrated,* that is, as *intrinsically* and *internally interactive* in a human being. Where human life is seen

---

824 Barth, *Church Dogmatics* III/4, 357 (my italics).

in terms of its biological or natural aspects, health is a descriptive, natural phenomenon: this is Christopher Boorse's viewpoint. Where human life is viewed as that which takes place in exchange and negotiation with societal and cultural demands, health, too, becomes a concept consistently negotiated and (almost entirely) defined by cultural values and demands: this is H. Tristram Engelhardt's position in "The Disease of Masturbation." And where the concern is with human life as the life of the individual in pursuit of certain ends, the end of happiness above all, then health becomes that which above all allows this pursuit. Such is Lennart Nordenfelt's argument, and these are, then, the fragments which key philosophers of the Anglo-American health debate propose.

As detailed earlier, Boorse's exclusive focus on the body is a too fragmentary basis for the clinical encounter. Conditioned by social, cultural, personal and moral factors, one may decide to suppress or deny the existence of bodily symptoms of dysfunctioning, even while experiencing a serious loss of functions. Within the Boors Ian account, it may be considered sufficient for the patient to hand over the dysfunctional body: the physician holds the (epistemological and technical) keys for its re-constitution. Yet what if treatment for a (functionally explained) tension headache fails, even where the patient has taken all medication and done all recommended exercises to release muscular tension, hence, to restore proper functioning? Subjective evaluations and explanations might play a role in both cause and cure of the tensions and these lie beyond a purely medical knowledge of functions.

In opposition to Boorse, H. Tristram Engelhardt in "The Disease of Masturbation" did not explicitly treat the reality of the organic body. His interest was to show the cultural dependency of medical concepts such as disease and health; he focused on the analysis and unmasking of how science controls human life through the translation of value judgements into seemingly neutral scientific explanation. His aim was to deconstruct the objective and uniform body of medical knowledge defended by Boorse.

Engelhardt's failure to acknowledge bodily reality left him with no foundation for a shared body of knowledge and treatment. Also, in focusing on cultural value judgements exclusively, he failed to see the importance of care for human individuality in the patient-physician encounter. For the clinical encounter to be successful it needs to include the action of taking care of the patient and his or her interpretation of dysfunction within the context of a personal life-story (as well as, of course, cultural, social and indeed political influences).

The advantage of Nordenfelt's interpretation of health was to allow medical practice and health care to be centred on the patient's individual needs, desires, and interpretations, as they are behind the initial impulse to seek the clinical encounter. The doctor is not the paternalist authority that administers treatment but more the enabler of life goals. Nordenfelt acknowledged that as gendered, bodily agents humans might pursue natural goals such as survival and reproduction, yet if so, then only due to their own autonomous choice of ends of action. Here, the question remains whether a common (social, cultural, political, or indeed natural) underpinning of health can be recognised in exclusively subjective and autono-

mous health interpretations. Are clinicians expected to react to individual demands only? It is difficult to see how medicine could practically be organised
such as to help humans to fulfil their many individual goals. Also, what are the
consequences of Nordenfelt's account for babies and young children with their
clearly limited abilities of formulating life goals? Is one to assume for them the
goal of survival as only vital life goal? Yet what is, then, the difference between
children and non-human animals?

Early Christian writers, and above all Augustine, show their views of health to
be bound up with their readings of both the nature *and meaning* of human existence. They explore human life in its natural, personal, spiritual, and social dimension. Augustine most explicitly ventures upon such exploration from the perspective of incarnation and resurrection. This allows him to start his interpretation of
health from the perspective of the unity of the material body (with its general
characteristics and its physiological variability) and the immaterial soul (as the
substrate of human relationship to God, the self, and others).

To refer to theology in the context of human life and health is not to say that
philosophy and/or today's natural and social sciences cannot indicate aspects of
personality, character or sociability as well as account for the interplay of body
and soul through logical inference, experience, introspection or empirical explanation of types of behaviour. What was sought here was something equating to
MacIntyre's lost context: a venture point through which what is today apparently
fragmentary and contradictory in these diverse accounts for health may be brought
together to inform medical practice and moral discourse.

Whilst as a "conceptual structure"[825] the body-soul union is found in Greek
philosophy, too, it is best understood not from logical inference or experience
alone but, as for Augustine, from the perspective of Christ's incarnation and resurrection.

This claim is at the centre of Oliver O'Donovan's 2002 article "Keeping Body
and Soul Together". It does not suffice to understand both the incarnation and
resurrection as a general affirmation of bodily life and of the good of the body,
O'Donovan argues. Rather, they constitute the "identification with a *body*"[826]
which through this identification is *someone's* body. As with Augustine, Christ's
resurrection is read by O'Donovan as showing to humans that the human body
will be taken up as the personalised body placed in a social network: whilst the
presence of every human being before the judgement seat of God *post resurrectionem* is that of a bodily individual with an irreplaceable story, this individual "is
itself an aspect of the presence of the whole human community."[827] O'Donovan
continues, "It is true that the resurrection grounds the eternal value of the individual. But it does so, not by backing the claim of the individual against the com-

825 O'Donovan, "Keeping Body and Soul Together", 46.
826 Ibid.
827 Ibid., 51.

munity."[828] It does so by developing the idea of the individual in identification with the body as a social being, which belongs to the community of people.

With regard to the body-soul union, O'Donovan emphasises, it is not the "conceptual structure *itself*" which differentiates New Testament anthropology from Platonic"[829] – for this structure is "plastic and adaptable"[830]– but that the resurrection became the centre of the earliest Christian proclamation. It was this that allowed the early church to "keep body and soul together" and that forbade developing a dual and fragmentary conception of humans as either species-typical bodies (Aristotle – and to an extent, Boorse) or self-sufficient, immortal souls (Plato – and to an extent, Nordenfelt).[831]

Augustine's understanding of human life allows for a view of the body as the "natural substrate"[832] of something as uniquely human as the freedom to act, widely acknowledged to pertain to the notion of personhood. He explores personal identity from within the doctrine of the *imago Dei*. It embraces ontological qualities which constitute the difference between humans and beasts such as reason, self-awareness, free will, and the capacity for meaningful decision-making.

Where human beings are recognised as personalised bodies, doctors may recognise their patients as interpreters of their actions and symptoms. Where they are recognised as bodily individuals, it makes sense that they consent or decline consent to treatment. Further, where humans are recognised as *intrinsically social* individuals constituted by their relationships to others, health professionals are able to recognise, for example, their patients' familial relationships, which are more complex than a description of biological related-ness can capture.[833]

Personal identity is not a natural category and cannot be described according to empirical observations, general appearances and measurable performance. It cannot be recognised from the distance of an experiment or in the planned observation of a behavioural test.[834] It does not belong to the world of facts. With Augustine, it can even be properly called *mysterious*. Beneath this, it may be called (as it is by O'Donovan) a hypothesis proved through human interaction, for it includes sociability: God's love directs humans to their fellow humans. Drawing on Augustine's reading of the personal or the soul in relation to the other, the physician always approaches the individual as placed in the midst of social relationships, as part of a community of people. Augustine's theology understands personhood, though ultimately mysterious, as always bodily, and sees the bodily individual within a community of people – a vision that was also at the forefront of

---

828 O'Donovan, "Keeping Body and Soul together", 51–52.

829 Ibid, 51.

830 Ibid., 46.

831 Ibid., 41.

832 O'Donovan, *Begotten or Made*, 5.

833 In genetic testing, where the knowledge of a patient's genes always includes knowledge of his or her parents', siblings', children's genes, the limits of informed, *individual* consent are reached, and forms of familial (or relational) consent need to be discussed.

834 Ibid., 59.

Basil's thinking where he stresses the importance of the community of care for medical healing.

Whilst it would be worthwhile exploring further the particular implications of the *personal* and *social* dimension of human life for health and medicine, I focus now on the aspect of being a personal *body*. I show how the value of bodily health motivates and limits medical action. Each of the following two sections starts with three theses on health, which are based on the central arguments of the preceding exegesis, above all the exegesis of Augustine's theological anthropology. The rhetoric of health as bodily repair and the argument of health's value as trumping the value of early human life as central features of the UK documents will be used to exemplify the practical implications of these theoretical claims for contemporary medicine.

6.2.2 The good of the body and the term repair

(1) The reality of bodily being and well-being originates in God who is the absolute good. (2) Therefore, the natural body is of value and to be valued. The pursuit of natural knowledge for the restoration of physical health is a worthy moral endeavour. (3) Due to the body-soul union, the natural body is personalised. As a consequence, medical knowledge needs to include physiological generalities and personal particularities; it does not repair natural mechanisms but seeks to cure the personalised body.

The body is a central characteristic of human life.

> "When we take off our clothes to have a bath, we confront something as natural, as given, as completely non-artifactual as anything in this universe: we confront our own bodily existence."[835]

The Christian belief in the resurrection affirms the body in its central position, and affirms it as good. It leads to a materialism that is inherent to any authentically Christian anthropology. A Christian materialism recognises the value of material existence whilst taking seriously the idea that humans are not simply flesh.

According to this materialism, humans are *biological* creatures: the *bodily* person and *personalised* body. Humans are *subjects* called by God. At the same time, in their constituted-ness as bodies, they are *objects* before God. A Christian materialism recognises the body in its always-particular nature. It rejects a naturalist species generalisation as can be derived from Aristotelianism. In recognising the good nature of the body it opposes an idealist spiritualisation (and individualisation) of humans, which goes back to Platonism.[836]

Against the background of the Christian monist view of human life, Augustine reflected on health as a good. In proclaiming the good of the body, beyond the Boorsian analysis, bodily health is not value-free in the Augustinian framework.

---

835 O'Donovan, *Begotten or Made*, 5.
836 O'Donovan, "Keeping Body and Soul Together", 41.

Yet such value, beyond Nordenfelt, is not the construct of a sovereign individual. Nor is it the construct of a controlling culture or society, as Engelhardt claimed. It originates in the Creator and his absolute goodness. It anticipates the fullness of life in the eschaton. Against the background of Augustine's reflection on sin, suffering and disease, health is a sign of God's vindication of life. Against Augustine's view of disease as divine punishment, health reflects the gift of salvation.

Whilst a Christian unified view of body and soul allows the defence of the material dimension of human life, a human being is never merely his or her brain, his or her heartbeat, his or her respirational functions. As O'Donovan concedes, one cannot engage with a human being "without the functioning brain, respiration and heartbeat." Yet, and this is the central point, what one meets and talks with is "not simply the sum of those functions, but another category of subject altogether."[837]

Based on the Augustinian position developed here and in the preceding, the human creature is bodily, material, universalisable in its functions and workings. Yet a full analysis and appreciation of the human body can never function in isolation to its personal-social nature and to its intrinsic value. A view of the body-soul union rooted in the resurrection holds that the bodily person and humanity in general exist in a social and political economy, which is determined by the loving social relations of the Trinity and the intrinsically social nature of humans made in its image.

Where a human being is not simply the sum of its bodily functions but a subject, the role of the physician who meets this objective subject (or subjective object) cannot be that of a technician or car mechanic. He or she is not simply "the man who stitches shirts", "the man who repairs old shoes"[838] or the man who weaves a shirt or makes new shoes[839] as Galen described the doctor's role. Following Augustine's anthropology, medicine is concerned with the patient as a being in union of body and soul, and not mere functional object. Hence, it cannot see somatic diseases *in abstraction* from that which makes human life in the diseased body particular and indeed meaningful. Where the vision of life developed by Augustine and pursued by theologians such as O'Donovan understands health as more than physiological functioning, medicine's role is not appropriately described by the term *repair* which is the term of preference in the 1998–2002 reports.

Apart from injuries, the target diseases of stem cell research include (mainly chronic) diseases or afflictions such as stroke, Parkinson's disease, Alzheimer's disease, Multiple Sclerosis or diabetes.[840] These are degenerative, cell-based diseases which are characterised by the misdirection or loss of regular cell functions which in turn leads to damaged tissues and/or to the loss of entire organs. The envisaged treatment for these diseases is described as the "*repair* of damaged tis-

---

837 O'Donovan, "Again: Who is a Person?", 126.
838 Galen, *To Thrasyboulos*, 67.
839 MacIntyre/Gorovitz, "Medical Fallibility", 75.
840 For a full account see DoH, *CMO Report*, Box 4, 18.

sue and organs."[841] The aim is "to develop tissue for use in the *repair* of failing organs, or for replacement of diseased or damaged tissues [...] to treat some rare but serious inherited disorders [...] to *repair* a woman's eggs."[842]

Commonly, *to repair* (Latin: *reparare*) is used with reference to non-living composite things or parts and structures. Etymologically, its meaning of 'to mend' describes the restoration of "a composite thing, structure etc. to good condition by renewal or replacement of decayed or damaged parts, or by fixing what has given way."[843] The Shakespearean use of repair with regards living objects in the sense of "to revive or recreate a person" or "to restore a person to a previous state" is obsolete in modern days English.[844] Whilst *repair* can indeed be the term of preference in the context of tissue or organs (that is, structures and parts of a composite thing), where the composite thing is not a material object solely but a human being composed of material body and immaterial soul other terms might describe more precisely what is or can be done to parts of this entity. For instance, *to recover* (Latin: *recuperare*) in its meaning of 'to get well again'[845] (that is, "to regain, acquire again, resume, return to: a quality, state, or condition; esp. health or strength; a faculty of body or mind or the use of this"[846]) would be an equally accurate term, also regarding organ functions. Further, *to recuperate* (Latin: *recuperare)* is used for the restoration both of material and immaterial things and for the recovery from ill health and exhaustion.[847]

Nevertheless this is not to say that *to repair* cannot be used appropriately in a medical context. However, where health is described *exclusively* as a result from repair work (as is the case in the 1998–2002 documents) what *might* be conjured up are images of the human being as a material object, possibly even a machine, which is in need of repair by a team of skilled mechanics. Should this be the case, the documents would be failing to acknowledge the significance of the body's intrinsic relation to human subjectivity. Is the human body in its biological mechanisms, in isolation of its individual and socio-personal dimension, the end of human embryonic stem cell research (and perhaps of medical research more generally) as critics of medicine such as Ivan Illich have warned since the 1970s?

Whilst the term *repair* might be problematic when it is used exclusively, it is at the same time intellectually legitimate in so far as it denotes the universalisable aspects of the body and of its parts (that which is material and objective about human beings, and which is the foundation of medicine as a science) and that therefore, for limited purposes, its use in reference to tissues (as in stem cell research) is certainly defensible. Yet an exclusive use is in risk of *reducing* humans to things; then, they are no longer able to grasp the transcendent character of their

---

841 DoH, *CMO Report*, ES 24, 9 (my italics) also 2, 16; 2.55, 29; 2.57, 29 and HoL, *Report*, 2.6, 11.
842 DoH, *CMO Report*, ES, 7 (my italics).
843 *The Oxford English Dictionary*, Vol. XIII, 628 (Oxford 1989).
844 Ibid.
845 Klein, *A Comprehensive Etymological Dictionary of the English Language,* Vol. II (1967).
846 *The Oxford English Dictionary*, Vol. XIII, 367 (Oxford 1989).
847 Ibid., 383.

existence as humans.[848] This would entail loosing an understanding of the aspects of human life which transcend the body so that "life itself becomes a mere 'thing'", which humans may claim as their exclusive property, completely subject to their control and manipulation.[849]

Drawing on coherent anthropology, medicine is able to (re-)integrate the physical and physiological generalities and intrinsic particularities of human life and move beyond an understanding of the body as a material object or thing. Certainly, we cannot engage with a human person "without the functioning brain, respiration and heartbeat" yet what we meet and talk with is "not simply the sum of those functions, but another category of subject altogether."[850] Such (re-)integration of particularity, then, links up to a restitution of the (traditional) role of the physician as adviser of the bodily *person* and healer of the personal *body*, of medicine as a science *and* art. For where the physician or researcher has a knowledge of the patient as a person, indeed they have a knowledge which is "typically particular rather than general, individual rather than collective, even (so far as it is practicable) *empathic* rather than intuitive."[851] An integrated vision of human life and health integrates scientific knowledge and personal care. On this basis, medicine looks at and seeks to sympathise with, to take care of the individual sufferer in her experience of dys-functioning within the wider context of her relationships and life goals.

Where humans view their bodily life as a mere objective functions, they become increasingly concerned with *doing*, with using all kinds of technology to apply to, and interfere with these functions and their different states.

Indeed, human naturalness and gendered-ness (and its contingency as experientially present in illness) appears more and more as an object at our disposal. Due to the advances of knowledge in the natural sciences and the possibilities this knowledge generates for medical treatment – especially when paired with recent technology developed by the engineering sciences – this object can be rejected, altered, enhanced. Birth and death, health and disease, "instead of being primary experiences demanding to be "lived", become things to be merely "possessed" or "rejected".[852]

Now, whilst Augustine recognised the natural reality of the body as an evaluated good, he never assumed that functioning alone was sufficient or indeed necessary for a happy and meaningful life. His recognition of health as a temporal and relative good indicates that our assessment of the pursuit of health in the context of particular medical practices needs to take account of other goods of life (namely, the goods of the soul) and to understand how bodily health relates to these goods, hence, how it ultimately relates to the goodness of God.

---

848 John Paul II, *Evangelium Vitae*, 39.
849 Ibid.
850 O'Donovan, "Again: Who is a person?", 126.
851 Toulmin, "Nature of the Physician's Understanding", 46 (my italics).
852 John Paul II, *Evangelium Vitae*, 39.

6.2.3 The value of health and the good of human life

Against the background of the prohibition of taking the life of post-fourteen day embryos, and indeed all human subjects in research, the move of connecting the end of potential health with the permission to take pre-fourteen day life needs to be looked at more closely. At least two points seem crucial in this context. They hinge on the often-debated question of the ontological status of the embryo, the related question of the respect we owe to embryos (as to human life more generally) and the wider question as to the value of goals of actions and the propositions such value judgements require respectively.

The two points are then: (1) how do we know whether or not the embryo is a person? Without being able to revisit here the extensive and controversial status debate, it will be discussed whether or not sense can be made of the notion of respect of human life in relation to the argument of twinning or genetic versus developmental identity, which is behind the fourteen-day-rule. Other criteria would be sentience, consciousness and so on, which cannot be discussed in the current context. (2) Apart from the status question, what is implicitly at work in the argumentation of the reports (CMO Report and HoL Select Committee reports above all) is a balance of values or moral weights linked up with a balance of probabilities, as Robert Song proposes in his 2003 article "To Be Willing to Kill What for All One Knows Is A Person Is to Be Willing to Kill a Person." In the reports, protecting the life of the pre-fourteen day embryo is given less moral weight compared with the weight given to the end of health of born humans (from babies to adults). The attribution of weight is related, Song shows, to probabilities – the probability of personhood and the probability of health benefits. According to the reports, the probability of the embryo's personhood is small, whereas the probability of health benefits of a number of sufferers is high. Against this, Song explains that where there is the possibility of personhood, the prohibition of killing human life makes the weighing up of human life against other goods (even where there are as worthy as the good of health) morally untenable. The underlying question, namely as to how we can know or determine the value of life and of health, and of both in relation to each other, is at the centre of this study and will be answered in engaging with philosophers and theologian of past and present. I address the two questions in turn.

Ad (1): The question as to the beginning of human life and the human, individual, personal, and value status of the human foetus and embryo has given rise to much debate and is discussed with great regularity in the context of artificial reproductive technologies and embryonic research.[853] Ultimately, it seems unlikely that it will ever be settled with a significant degree of unanimity or cer-

853 For a summary of the debate see for instance Ford, *When Did I Begin? Conception of the Human Individual in History, Philosophy, and Science* (Cambridge, 1988) and Holland/Lebacqz/Zoloth, *The Human Embryonic Stem Cell Debate: Science, Ethics, and Public Policy* (Cambridge, MA 2001). Two opposing views of embryonic life are for instance Singer/Kuhse (ed): *Embryo Experimentation* (Cambridge, 1990) and Roman Catholic arguments based on Thomas Aquinas, *Summa Theologiae*, 111, Q. 16.

tainty.[854] Yet the issue of the ontological status of the embryo is clearly critical as it is connected with the issue of *respect* owed to embryos and the practical implications of such respect – i.e. the question whether or not the showing of respect is compatible with destroying embryos in the process of reproductive treatment or research.

As mentioned above, many (and not only theologians) hold that the human individual is already formed in the zygote since the human adult develops from the zygote in a continuous and coordinated biological process. The same zygote appears to organise itself into an embryo (foetus, infant, child, adult) without ceasing to be substantially the same living individual. This seems to indicate that the zygote is an *actual* human being or individual, not just a *potential* human individual. Also, the genetic identity of the adult is practically the same as that of the zygote. On these grounds it is then possible to believe that 'the immaterial soul' subsists 'zygotically' as it were, though its immateriality prohibits by definition empirical evidence to verify this.

Others, such as the voices present in the 1998–2002 reports, emphasise the fact that identical twins (that is, *two* individuals) may be formed from the zygote and that therefore a (that is, *one single*) human individual cannot be seen as in continuation with the zygote. The potency for identical twinning is lost after the primitive streak stage, post-fourteen days, when differentiation has progressed to the point of forming a definitive individual. While the first group argues for the zygote as a human individual on grounds of genetic identity, the second argues against it on grounds of developmental identity.[855] Even though genetic individuality exists from the moment of fertilisation, the latter say, developmental *individuality* only exists post-fourteen days, hence, the fourteen days cut-off point for research on embryos.

Yet twinning is nothing else but this: a possibility. Indeed, there might (or might not) be two personal histories developing out of one genetical identity. What does this demonstrate with regard to the individuality of the zygote? Oliver O'Donovan argues that in the end the possibility of twinning only shows that even though genetic individuality "seems to provide the indication of the beginning of a new personal history at conception"[856] it is not to be identified with personal individuality. "To observe a gene is not to observe a person. What genetics can do is to show us an *appearance* of a human being which has decisive continuities with late appearances."[857] For O'Donovan it does not seem to be clear how the fact that one genetically individual embryo might develop into two persons morally justifies its destruction for research purposes. Rather the opposite: whilst it does *not*

---

854 Cf. Song, "To Be Willing to Kill", 102 – "Indeed to claim that there must be no doubt at all, that it must be absolutely certain that the embryo is not a person before one could research on it, would require a level of certainty which is arguably not even in principle attainable by human beings".

855 Cf. McCormick, "Who or What is the Pre-embryo?" (1991).

856 O'Donovan, *Begotten or Made*, 56.

857 Ibid., 51.

show that this entity is devoid of personhood, what it does show is that, indeed, *two* individual persons may develop.

Independent of the difficulties of settling the question of the ontological status of the embryo on biological grounds, approaches to this question as of the value of human life more generally are shaped by a variety of intellectual, cultural or historical presuppositions and beliefs. In late Antiquity the value of human life depended on a human being's ability to contribute towards the societal good, a view which was to the disadvantage not only of babies and children but also women and slaves. Social rankings, as much as biological stages, underlie the attribution of value; indeed, a human being's value in Antiquity was largely defined as social value; a person was seen to be of value in view of his or her potential to contribute both materially and through its acquired virtues to the good of the family and of society.

Children generally were considered of value only in so far as they had the potential of making virtuous contribution to the public good once they had reached adulthood. "It was almost universally held in antiquity that a child has no intrinsic right to life in virtue of being born. What mattered was being adopted into a family or some other institution of the society."[858] The exposure of *both* healthy and defective newborns was widely practiced both in Classical Greece and Rome. Whilst the former were exposed for economic reasons and population control, the latter were left to die for social and eugenic benefits to society.

In relation to the appreciation of human life as of intrinsic value, the advent of Christianity marked a turning point in late Antiquity: early Christian theologians give testimony of a different attitude towards human life and society from beginning to end (whereby often 'the beginning' refers to the moment of conception, hence, the almost unanimous condemnation of abortive practices amongst early Christianity) and set examples of social practices that paved the way for public institutions of charity for the socially excluded as per the universality of the Kingdom of God (as opposed to the Greek polis). They reacted to, and often against, the dominant attitudes towards the body and life more generally as of bearing value in terms of its contributions to the public good. They attacked the practice of exposure of not only but also defective newborns. They showed little interest in particular disabilities or diseases, and if so (as in the case of leprosy) then in relation to social exclusion more generally. And while the Church Fathers of the late third and fourth century showed little, if no, theoretical interest in the origin or moral nature of physical differences, they were adamant to recommend pastoral care and philanthropy as examples of good agency given in the New Testament in reaction to social exclusion and reflective of the Kingdom of God.

Ad (2): I now move on to discuss the connection between value and probabilities, between the value of the embryo and its possibility of personhood on the one hand, and the value of research and its possibility for benefiting large numbers of patients on the other.

---

858 Rist, *Human Value*, 141.

In his 2003 article "To Be Willing to Kill What for All One Knows Is A Person Is to Be Willing to Kill a Person" Robert Song looks at the question of the ontology of the human embryo in response to the treatment of the question given by the HoL Select Committee. He focuses on the argument whether or not the embryo should be given the benefit of the doubt in a situation where proofs as to its personhood or non-personhood are equally difficult to provide. Usually, critics of embryonic research who appeal to it in favour of the embryo employ benefit of the doubt arguments but, as he claims, the significance of this argument "has been misunderstood by both its advocates and its critics."[859]

As Song illustrates, both advocates and critics of the argument refer to a model of balancing scales when arguing their positions. Advocates usually argue that where all substantive arguments have failed to produce a conclusion as regards the embryo's personhood, the embryo should be given the benefit of the doubt. "The implicit model behind the appeal to benefit of the doubt is a balance of probabilities, where the evenly-balanced scales will be tipped in favour of the embryo once this argument is added to the pan."[860] And – as has been shown in the analysis of the 1998–2002 reports – critics of the argument explicitly refer to a model of scales, too, when they speak about the weighing up probabilities. In Song's words,

> "The embryo being a person acts as a kind of reducing factor, such that the possibility of killing someone should be given a fraction of the weight that would be attributed to actually killing someone. Once that is accepted, the possibility of developing therapies for serious and common diseases then outweighs the now rather abstract notion of destroying a possible person."[861]

A claim central to Song's article is that both advocates and critics of embryonic research, in referring to a balance of probabilities, have lost the *argumentative force* which is *contained in the possibility that in the process of such research someone might be killed*. Only where the force of this possibility is taken seriously, are we able to see that the moral weights of the balancing scales are wrongly calibrated, and hence, that the balance model itself becomes morally untenable.

And it is with this turn that Song's article becomes of direct relevance to the question before us, namely of weighing up the good of embryonic life and the good of health, and with a view to this study as a whole, to the question of how to attribute value to human life (embryonic life more particularly) and health.

Where we refer to the model of scales in trying to solve the moral dilemma of using embryos in research, Song argues that rather than attributing "a measure of respect" (that is, small weight) to the embryo on grounds of its potential personhood we should attribute a full degree of respect (or greatest weight). Song's point here is that whilst we cannot know or say with reasonable[862] certainty whether or

---

859 Song, "To Be Willing to Kill", 98.
860 Ibid.
861 Ibid.
862 Song is keen to underline that in embryonic research (as in all biomedical research using living beings) it is not a question of *no doubt at all* as to the embryo's status but of being

not embryos are persons, such uncertainty does not tell us anything about their actual state. Whilst we can say that we cannot *demonstrate* whether or not they are persons, *there always remains the possibility that they are*. Hence, we always face the risk that where we take away an embryo's life in the process of research, we take away a person's life – which then goes against the prohibition of killing.

Now, as Song points out, a difficulty in the context of embryo research is that "the merely possible personhood of the embryo may seem *abstract or theoretical* in comparison with the *ostensibly concrete hopes for clinical treatments* derived from embryonic stem cell research."[863] So, in a balance where possible clinical treatment of actual, living persons and the intangible possibility of an embryo's personhood are weighed up against each other, the first seems concrete and tangible, the latter abstract and somewhat unrelated to our lives.

Whilst indeed the concrete often rules over the abstract mostly in our intuitive decision making, in the reports, which strive for reasonable not intuitive morality, 'the concrete' and 'the abstract' seem to be replaced by a language of mathematical calculation which is behind the balancing of 'greater' and 'lesser weights'. That which is concrete (namely health benefits for sufferers who we might *be* or *know* and *have relationships with*) is given greater weight; that which is abstract (namely the nameless pre-fourteen day embryos whose personhood exists, if at all, invisibly or mysteriously and who we can *never* be) is attributed lesser weight. This is not to say that the pre-fourteen day embryo has no moral weight – in all three reports *early* embryonic life is described as deserving a measure of respect – yet its life is not worthy enough to prohibit it being ended for the health benefits of suffering human subjects.

Now, for Song in attributing small weight to the embryo the reports are mistaken: where the possibility exists that the embryo has its life at stake (and such possibility exists even when we take seriously arguments such as twinning, consciousness and so on) what we are weighing up is not 'probably-*not*-personal-life' and 'probably-health' but 'possibly-personal-life' and 'possibly-health'. And this is why Song argues that, where personal life is possibly at stake, its weighing up against other goods is morally untenable: where life *might be* present, we are bound by the prohibition against killing to act as if it *is* present.[864]

To reject the balancing of life against other goods such as the good of health does not equal a rejection of the good of health. What it says is that life is a good *beyond all other goods* in that it is the condition for all other goods and whilst in moral decision making we are constantly involved in balancing and outweighing values and ends, it says that the good of life cannot be outweighed by, or used in the service of, the good of health.

In "To Be Willing to Kill" Song has provided an argument for the protection of the embryo which bears directly on legal discourse as to the rights to be ac-

---

satisfied beyond *reasonable doubt* that embryos do not have a status that should protect them from lethal harm.

863 Song, "To Be Willing to Kill", 101 (my italics).
864 Ibid.

corded to the embryo. He pointed out that those who support the use of embryos in research need to show beyond reasonable doubt that the embryo is *not* a person; those who hold that reasonable doubt does obtain, will be against it. He stressed the importance of recognising that what is required is not absolute certainty *beyond doubt at all* but certainty *beyond reasonable doubt* – for, indeed, the former would have bizarre implications as regards lethal research on animals, including laboratory animals such as fruit-flies and nematode worms.

Song highlighted the impossibility of demonstrating with certainty that embryos are persons. In a similar vein, Oliver O'Donovan underlines in his discussion of personhood in *Begotten or Made* that the question of when, particularly, personhood begins is *not* susceptible to straightforward, factual answers. He explains that human personhood is no natural (biological, genetic) category that can be described according to empirical or statistical observations, general appearances and measurable performance. To understand personality as the ways in which the human embryo, the child, the adult is *personal* requires another mode of deliberation, one "which discerns the hypostasis behind the appearances."[865] Such a mode a deliberation might have as its parameters engagement, commitment and love, that is, it can only be discovered "through interaction and commitment that this human being is irreplaceable."[866] O'Donovan eludes this idea not with reference to the objectivity of the laboratory, but with a story: that of the Good Samaritan.

> "'Who is my neighbour?' asked the lawyer of Jesus. 'Who', Jesus asked in reply, 'proved neighbour to the man who fell among thieves?'" To discern my neighbour, I have first to 'prove' neighbour to him. To perceive a brother or a sister, I have first to act in a brotherly way. To know a person, I have first to accept him as such in personal interaction. Quite different from this is all experimental knowledge, which is acquired by achieving a masterful distance on its object in testing and proof. Such knowledge cannot be knowledge of the hidden, of that which underlies appearances. It looks for appearances, and it finds appearances."[867]

This story tells us, then, that personhood cannot be recognised from the distance of an experiment or in the planed observation of a behavioural test. It is a hypothesis proved through neighbourly interaction. Neighbourly interaction is not posterior, based upon the results of scientific testing which first determines whether the other demands such respect.

6.2.4 The good of health – an imperative for medicine?

(1) Bodily health is a temporal good: human life is limited by death. (2) The value of bodily health has its cause in God's absolute goodness. In this, it is a good relative to God's goodness; it is not an absolute value to which God, too, would have to bow. (3) Due to the body-soul union the value of bodily health needs to be

865 O'Donovan, *Begotten or Made*, 57.
866 Ibid., 59.
867 Ibid., 60.

*viewed in relation to the other goods given to humans by God, such as the good of
happiness or joy. Happiness and joy are lived in the body but stem from the soul's
orientation towards God. As a consequence, bodily health is only one aspect of
human well-being or fulfilment, and it is subordinated to the goods of the soul.*

Despite exciting medical advances and promising novel therapies, bodily health
remains a fugitive good: death is interwoven with the organic, historical substance
of human life. For Augustine, human mortality is God's punishment for the
disobedience for which the myth of Genesis accounts. Due to the finitude of
existence, where physicians seek cures they also learn the limits of their craft and
that "the sheer particularity of the patient's illness often defies the best knowledge
and skill."[868] Their desire to know, to probe nature, and to fight diseases may be
seen as an expression of the genuinely human attempt to deal with human
mortality. Yet death will be overcome in the eschatological future only, not
through medical endeavours, not even the most sophisticated and technologically
advanced. Notwithstanding the temporal nature of bodily health, where it is understood
as serving human existence in its bodily functions and personal life goals,[869] the
relief of suffering is of great moral importance. Human embryonic stem cell research indeed may restore health and relieve suffering. Such health gains may be a
sign of God's care, and indicative of his salvation. They may be celebrated.

Yet at the same time, as the early Christian writers engaged with in the preceding underlined, health is always only *one* desideratum of a truly good, fulfilled
and meaningful human life. They considered bodily health of secondary importance when compared with spiritual well-being. And they emphasised that medicine may always also be used for sinful ends, that is, ends disproportionate *to the
order established by God as love.* Situating bodily health and medical action
within this order means that they are goods to be viewed in light of this love.

Such a view does not minimise the value of health and of medicine's pursuit
of healing. Based on Augustine's reading of the body-soul union within the order
of salvific love, the pursuit of bodily health can indeed trump other human goods:
it reflects God's will for humans to be healthy. Whilst it is never an absolute, nor
even a primary imperative,

> "At a few times and places it may seem imperative; at many times and places it is desirable;
> in some times and places, because we judge other, competing goods to be even more funda-
> mental to human life, it may be neither imperative nor desirable."[870]

Humans must oppose suffering as best as they can, that is, within the limits appropriate to human life. However, assessing the importance of bodily health in
relation to other "competing" goods (above all the goods of the social and individual soul) might lead to the recognition that in certain circumstances bodily
health does not need to be pursued, for it does not lead to fullness of life. Lasting

---

868 Hauerwas, "Salvation and Health", 220.
869 Barth, *Church Dogmatics* III/4, 357 (my italics).
870 Meilaender, http://www.bioethics.gov/background/meilaenderpaper.html, last accessed 01/-
     2010.

health and happiness lie in God's love and wisdom, which, as Christ's life and death showed, are mysteriously present *in particular* in suffering and pain.

According to the UK documents looked at in chapter two, in human embryonic stem cell research the competing goods to be weighed up are the good of potential health and the value of the early embryo's life. It has been discussed why it does not make sense morally to oppose the value of health benefits and the value of early life in this way. Based on the anthropology explored throughout this study, we may conclude that in the early embryo personhood is at least as mysteriously present and bound up with the material substrate of life as it is in any other human being. Where the early embryo is viewed thus, it does not make sense to attribute to it "special status and value" and to weigh its value up against the value of potential health benefits.

Further, where one draws on Augustine's anthropology in the context of early embryo research, one is directed again to his hierarchical view of body and soul. It includes the subordination of the goods of the body to those of the soul. Happiness is one of the soul's goods; it is gained where the soul stretches out and orients itself towards God. "If we follow after Him, we live well; if we reach Him, we live not only well, but happily."[871] Happiness is valued higher than physical health, and what is more, can be realised even where humans experience disease and pain.

This subordination of the body to the soul, then, limits medicine's imperative of cure. It does not deny the moral importance of the relief of suffering: in situating bodily health and medical action within God's redemptive action, they are both good. Bodily health may signify God's restoring grace present in this world: bodily health as well as happiness and joy reflect eternal health, joy and happiness, which are granted in the fullness of salvation. Health anticipates complete and full well-being in body and soul. Yet, notwithstanding the affirmation of bodily health and medicine, God's love as it revealed itself as particularly present in suffering and pain, revealed bodily health as only *one* desideratum of a truly good, fulfilled and meaningful human life.

6.3 CONCLUDING REMARKS

Against the background of the preceding exegesis of philosophical and theological approaches to the concept of health, the understanding of health I proposed in the section above is grounded in the context of human life lived in the indissoluble union of the natural, and the personal-social. Health therefore is neither physical (which includes *the mental* in as much as it is related to states of the brain) nor psychical health alone. Against Engelhardt, it is held that there is such a thing as organic health beyond it being an arbitrary, even tyrannical social construct. But, against Boorse, objective organic health is not conceived as impersonal and value-

---

871 Augustine, *The Way of Life*, 6, 10.

free. Embodied humanity refuses the description of the healthy body as a thing that becomes the passive object of science.

Yet health's value, against Nordenfelt, is not the construct of the sovereign and abstract individual, anymore than of a controlling society; it is theologically derived and rooted in God's loving relationship to humans.

Where the union of body and soul is taken seriously, in particular the body's intrinsic orientation towards God via the soul, health is not a good or end in itself. Moral priority is attributed to humanity's orientation towards God's love pursued in fellowship with other humans and in engagement with creation as a whole. Where health is not an end in itself but points to, and serves, this ultimate end of life, humans are freed from the need to strive for health for its own sake or for their *selves* independent of *the other*, for better work, or for greater market efficiency.

Having its place in the context of human life, the understanding of health I propose with Augustine does not aim at the physician or clinician exclusively.

It speaks to the physician *and* the patient. It addresses human persons – not societies or populations. Nor does it aim to be a medical model without, however, positing itself outside the practical sphere of medicine. It seeks to contextualise medicine's role with the ultimate source of all healing which also is the measure of all things: God's love. This proposition is directed at medicine in that medicine does its greatest service to humans where it *assists* in accomplishing the goals of life proposed by this love.

The understanding of health developed in critical engagement with contemporary (Anglo-American) philosophy of medicine, patristic writers (above all Augustine) as well as contemporary theologians and bioethicists recognises the natural and good reality of the body and integrates natural and medical contributions to healing. Yet it does not assume that natural health was sufficient and indeed necessary for a happy and meaningful life, for human flourishing. It recognises the socio-personal dimension of human life and is able to integrate sociological, psychological, anthropological and philosophical approaches to health. However, it can neither be uncritical in its use of, and is not exhausted in, any one of these approaches. Neither of them is adequate on their own, where they stand independently from the meaning of human life that has been disclosed in the life and resurrection of Jesus Christ.

SELECTED BIBLIOGRAPHY

Amundsen, D.W., "Medicine and Faith in Early Christianity", in: *Bulletin of the History of Medicine*, 56 (1982), 326–350.

Amundsen, D.W., "Tatian's 'Rejection' of Medicine in the Second Century", in: *Ancient Medicine in Its Socio-Cultural Context*, ed. Van der Eijk/Horstmanshoff/Schrijvers (Amsterdam, 1995), 377–392.

Amundsen, D.W., "Body, Soul, and Physician", in: *Medicine, Society and Faith in the Ancient and Medieval Worlds*, ed. Amundsen (London/New York, 1996), 1–30.

Amundsen, D.W., *Medicine, Society and Faith in the Ancient and Medieval Worlds* (London/New York, 1996).

Amundsen, D.W., *Caring and Curing. Health and Medicine in the Western Religious Traditions* (London/New York, 1998).

Anderson, J.F., *St. Augustine and Being: a Metaphysical Essay* (The Hague, 1965).

Arbesmann, R., "Christ the *Medicus Humilis* in St. Augustine", in: *Augustinus Magister: Congrès International Augustinian, Paris, 21-24 September 1954. Communications*, 1 (1954), 623–630.

Aristotle, *Metaphysics*, trans. H. Lawson-Tancred (London, 1998).

Aristotle, *On the Soul*, trans. H. Lawson-Tancred (London, 1986).

Aristotle, *The Nicomachean Ethics*, trans. D. Ross (Oxford, 1998).

Armstrong, A.H., *Plotinian and Christian Studies* (London, 1979).

Armstrong, A.H./Markus, R.A., *Christian Faith and Greek Philosophy* (London, 1960).

Armstrong, D., *A Materialist Theory of the Mind* (London, 1968).

Armstrong, D., *The Mind-Body Problem. An Opinionated Introduction* (Colorado/Oxford, 1999).

Arnold, D.W.H./Bright, P., *De Doctrina Christiana. A Classic of Western Culture* (Notre Dame/London, 1995).

Aronowitz, R.A., *Making Sense of Illness: Science, Society and Disease* (Cambridge, 1998).

Augustine, *Expositions of the Psalms, Psalms 1–32*, trans. M. Bounding O.S.B., in: The Works of St. Augustine: A Translation for the 21st Century, ed. J.E. Roselle, III/15 (New York, 2000).

Augustine, *Expositions of the Psalms, Psalms 33–50*, trans. M. Bounding O.S.B., in: The Works of St. Augustine: A Translation for the 21st Century, ed. J.E. Roselle, III/16 (New York, 2001).

Augustine, *Expositions of the Psalms, Psalms 51–72*, trans. M. Bounding O.S.B., in: The Works of St. Augustine: A Translation for the 21st Century, ed. J.E. Roselle, III/17 (New York, 2001).

Augustine, *Expositions of the Psalms, Psalms 73–98*, trans. M. Bounding O.S.B., in: The Works of St. Augustine: A Translation for the 21st Century, ed. J.E. Roselle, III/18 (New York, 2002).

Augustine, *Letters 1–82*, trans. Sr. Wilfrid Parsons, in: The Fathers of the Church, 12 (Washington, 1951).

Augustine, *Letters 100–155*, trans. R. Teske S.J., in: The Works of St. Augustine: A Translation for the 21st Century, ed. B. Ramsey, II/2 (New York, 2003).

Augustine, *The City of God Against the Pagans*, trans. R.W. Dyson (Cambridge, 1998).

Augustine, *The Confessions*, trans. H. Chadwick (Oxford, 1992).

Augustine, *The Literal Meaning of Genesis*, trans. E. Hill O.P., in: The Works of St. Augustine: A Translation for the 21st Century, ed. J.E. Roselle, I/13 (New York, 2002).

Augustine, *The Trinity*, trans. S. McKenna C.SS.R, in: The Fathers of the Church, 45 (Washington, 1981).

Augustine, *The Way of Life of the Catholic Church*, trans. D.A. Gallagher/I.J. Gallagher, in: The Fathers of the Church, 56 (Washington, 1966).

Banner, M., *Christian Ethics and Contemporary Moral Problems* (Cambridge, 1999).

Banner, M., *A Brief History of Christian Ethics* (Cambridge, 2010).

Bardy, G., "Saint Augustine et les medicines", in: *L'Année Theologique Augustienne*, 47/48 (1953), 327–346.

Barnes, J., "Galen on Logic and Therapy", in: Kudlien, F./Dorling, R.J.: *Galen's Method of Healing. Proceedings of the 1982 Galen Symposium* (Leiden/New York, 1991), 50–102.

Barth, K., *Church Dogmatics*, II: 2, trans. G. Bromiley et al. (Edinburgh, 1957).

Barth, K., *Church Dogmatics*, III: 2, trans. H. Knight et al. (Edinburgh, 1960).

Barth, K., *Church Dogmatics* III: 4, trans. A.T. Mackay et al. (Edinburgh, 1961).

Basil the Great, *Ascetical Works*, trans. Sr. M. Monica Wagner, in: The Fathers of the Church, 9 (Washington, 1950).

Beck, M., *Seele und Krankheit: Psychosomatische Medizin und theologische Anthropologie* (Paderborn, 2000).

Beck, M., *Hippokrates am Scheideweg* (Paderborn, 2001).

Bergner, G.B., "Early Christianity as a Religion of Healing", in: *Bulletin of the History of Medicine*, 66 (1992), 1–15.

Berlin-Brandenburg Academy of the Sciences (BBAW), *Zweiter Gentechnologiebericht* (Berlin, 2010).

Bonhoeffer, D., *Ethics*, ed. E. Bethge, transl. N.H. Smith (London, 1955).

Bonner, G., *St Augustine of Hippo: Life and Controversies* (London, 1963).

Bonner, G., *Saint Augustine and the Augustinian Tradition* (Villanova, 1972).

Bonner, G., "Contra Julianum", in: *Augustine Through the Ages: An Encyclopaedia*, ed. A.D. Fitzgerald (Grand Rapids/Cambridge, 1999), 480–481.

Boorse, C., "On the Distinction Between Disease and Illness", in: *Philosophy and Public Affairs*, 5/1 (1975), 49–68.

Boorse, C., "What a Theory of Mental Health Should Be", in: *Journal of Theory of Social Behaviour*, 6/1 (1976), 61–84.

Boorse, C., "Health as a Theoretical Concept", in: *Philosophy of Science*, 44 (1977), 542–573.

Brachtendorf, J., *Die Struktur des menschlichen Geistes nach Augustinus. Selbstreflexion und Erkenntnis Gottes in "De Trinitatis"* (Hamburg, 2000).

Brandt, R.B., *A Theory of the Good and the Right* (Oxford, 1979).

Breck, J., *Scripture in Tradition. The Bible and its Interpretation in the Orthodox Church* (New York, 2001).

Brown, P., *Augustine of Hippo: A Biography* (London, 1967).

Brown, P., *The Cult of the Saints: Its Rise and Function in Latin Christianity* (London, 1981).

Brown, P., *Body and Society: Men, Women, and Sexual Renunciation in Early Christianity* (London, 1989).

Brown, R.F., "The First Evil Will Must Be Incomprehensible: A Critique of Augustine", in: *Journal of the American Academy of Religion*, 46/3 (1978), 315–329.

Burnaby, J., *Amor Dei: A Study of the Religion of St. Augustine* (London, 1938).

Burns, C.R., "The naturals: A Paradox in the Western Concept of Health", in: *The Journal of Medicine and Philosophy*, 1/3 (1976), 202–211.

Burns, J.P., "Grace", in: *Augustine through the Ages: An Encyclopaedia*, ed. A.D. Fitzgerald (Grand Rapids/Cambridge, 1999), 391–398.

Busch, E., *Die große Leidenschaft. Einführung in die Theologie Karl Barths* (Darmstadt, 2001).

Callahan, D., "The WHO Definition of 'Health'", in: *Hastings Center Report*, 1/3 (1973), 77–87.

Callahan, D., "The Puzzle of Profound Respect", in: *Hastings Center Report*, 25/1 (1995), 39–40.

Camus, A., *La Peste* (Paris, 1947).

Camus, A., *The Plague*, trans. S. Gilbert (London, 1948).

Canguilhem, G., *The Normal and the Pathological*, trans. C.R. Fawcett (New York, 1989).

Carter, R.B., *Descartes' Medical Philosophy: The Organic Solution to the Mind-Body Problem* (London/Baltimore, 1983).

Chadwick, H., *Early Christian Thought and the Classical Tradition: Studies in Justin, Clement and Origen* (Oxford, 1996).

Changeux, J-P./Ricoeur, P., *What Makes us Think? A Neuroscientist and a Philosopher Argue About Ethics, Human Nature and the Brain* (Princeton, N.J./Oxford, 2000).

Christian, W.A., "The Creation of the World", in: *A Companion to the Study of St. Augustine*, ed. R.W. Battenhouse (Oxford, 1955), 315–342.

Cibelli, J.B. et al., "Somatic Cell Nuclear Transfer in Humans: Pronuclear and Early Embryonic Development", in: *Journal of Regenerative Medicine*, 2 (2001), 25–31.

Clark, M.T., "Irenaeus", in: *Augustine Through the Ages: An Encyclopaedia*, ed. A.D. Fitzgerald (Grand Rapids/Cambridge, 1999), 456–457.

The Council of Europe, *Convention on Human Rights and Biomedicine* (1997), http://conventions.coe.int/treaty/en/treaties/html/168.htm.

Cochrane, C.N., *Christianity and Classical Culture* (Oxford, 1940).

Condi, M.L., "The Basics about Stem Cells", in: *First Things*, 119 (2002), 30–39.

Courtès, J., "Saint Augustine et la medicine", in: *Augustinus Magister: Congrès International Augustinien, Paris, 21-24 September 1954. Communications*, 1 (1954), 43–52.

Coyle, J.K., "Mani, Manicheism", in: *Augustine Through the Ages: An Encyclopedia*, ed. A.D. Fitzgerald (Grand Rapids/Cambridge, 1999), 520–525.

Cramer, W., *Der Geist Gottes und des Menschen in frühsyrischer Theologie* (1979).

Damjanow, I./Lindner, J., *Anderson's Pathology* (New York, 1996).

Dawson, G.G., *Healing: Pagan and Christian* (London, 1935).

Declaration Of Helsinki, confirmed by the 35th World Medical Assembly, Venice, Italy, October 1983 (1964), http://bmj.bmjjournals.com/cgi/content/full/313/7070/1448/a.

Department of Health, *Stem Cell Research: Medical Progress with Responsibility. A Report from the Chief Medical Officer's Expert Group Reviewing the Potential of Developments in Stem Cell Research and Cell Nuclear Replacement to Benefit Human Health* (London, 2000).

Department of Health, *Government's Response to the Recommendations Made in the Chief Medical Officer's Expert Group Report 'Stem Cell Research: Medical Progress with Responsibility'* (London, 2000).

Descartes, R., *Meditations on First Philosophy*, trans. E.S. Haldane/G.R.T. Ross, in: Key Philosophical Writings (Herefordshire, 1997).

Diepgen, P., "Der Kirchenlehrer Augustin und die Anatomie im Mittelalter", in: *Centaurus*, 1/1 (1950), 206–211.

D'Irsay, S., "Christian Medicine and Science in the Third Century", in: *Journal of Religion*, 10 (1930), 515–544.

Dodds, E.R., *Pagans and Christians in an Age of Anxiety* (Cambridge, 1965).

Doerflinger, R.M., "The Ethics of Funding Embryonic Stem Cell Research: A Catholic Viewpoint, in: *Kennedy Institute of Ethics Journal*, 9/2 (1999), 137–150.

Duncan, G., "Mind-Body Dualism and the Biopsychosocial Model of Pain: What Did Descartes Really Say?", in: *The Journal of Medicine and Philosophy*, 25/4 (2000), 485–513.

Edelstein, E.J./Edelstein, L., *Asclepius*, 2 Vol. (Baltimore, 1945).

Edwards, M.J., "Neoplatonism", in: *Augustine Through the Ages: An Encyclopaedia*, ed. A.D. Fitzgerald (Grand Rapids/Cambridge, 1999), 588–591.

Eijkenboom, P.C., *Het Christus-Medicusmotief in de Preen van Sint Augustinus* (Rotterdam, 1960).

Elze, M., *Tatian und seine Theologie*, in: Forschungen zur Kirchen- und Dogmengeschichte, 9 (1960).

Engel, G.L., "The Need for a New Medical Model: A Challenge for Biomedicine", in: *Science*, 196/4286 (1977), 129–136.

Engelhardt, H.T., Jr., "The Disease of Masturbation: Values and the Concept of Disease", in: *The Bulletin of the History of Medicine*, 48/2 (1974), 234–248.

Engelhardt, H.T., Jr./Spicker, S.F. (eds.), *Evaluation and Explanation in the Biomedical Sciences: Proceedings of the 1. Transdisciplinary Symposium on Philosophy and Medicine, Held at Galveston, May 9–11, 1974*, Philosophy and Medicine (Dordrecht, 1975).

Engelhardt, H.T., Jr., "The Concepts of Health and Disease", in: *Evaluation and Explanation in the Biomedical Sciences: Proceedings of the 1. Transdisciplinary Symposium on Philosophy and Medicine, Held at Galveston, May 9–11, 1974*, Philosophy and Medicine (Dordrecht, 1975), 125–141.

Engelhardt, H.T., Jr., "Ideology and Aetiology", in: *The Journal of Medicine and Philosophy*, 1/3 (1976), 256–268.

Engelhardt, H.T., Jr., *The Foundations of Christian Bioethics* (Amsterdam, 2000).

Engelhardt, H.T., Jr., *The Philosophy of Medicine. Framing the Field*, Philosophy and Medicine (Dordrecht, 2000).

Engels, E.-M., "Der moralische Status von Embryonen und Feten - Forschung, Diagnose, Schwangerschaftsabbruch", in: *Ethik in der Humangenetik*, ed. Mieth, D./Düwell, M. (Tübingen/Basel, 1998), 271–301.

Evans, G.R., *Augustine on Evil* (Cambridge, 1982).

Fabrega, H., "Concepts of Disease: Logical Features and Social Implications", in: *Perspectives in Biology and Medicine*, 15 (1972), 583–616.

Fedoryka, K., "Health as a Normative Concept: Towards a New Conceptual Framework", in: *The Journal of Medicine and Philosophy*, 22/2 (1997), 143–160.

Ferguson, E., *Christian Life, Ethics, Morality and Discipline in the Early Church* (1993).

Ford, N.M., *When Did I Begin? Conception of the Human Individual in History, Philosophy, and Science* (Cambridge, 1988).

Foster, C., "Bentham on the Slippery Slope? Discussing Embryo Research in Britain's Parliament and Churches", in: *Zeitschrift Evangelische Ethik*, 46 (2002), 61–65.

Foucault, M., *The Birth of the Clinic: An Archaeology of Medical Perception*, trans. A.M. Sheridan Smith (New York, 1973).

Fox, M.M., *The Life and Times of St. Basil the Great As Revealed in his Works* (Washington, 1939).

Frede, M., "On Galen's Epistemology", in: *Galen. Problems and Prospects*, ed. V. Nutton (London, 1981), 65–86.

Frede, M., *Essays in Ancient Philosophy* (Oxford, 1987).

Frend, W.H.C., *The Donatist Church. A Movement of Protest in Roman North Africa* (Oxford, 1985).

Frings, H.-J., *Medizin und Arzt bei den griechischen Kirchenvätern bis Chrysostomos*. PhD-thesis (Bonn, 1959).

Frost. E., *Christian Healing: A Consideration of the Place of Spiritual Healing in the Church of To-day in the Light of the Doctrine and Practice of the Anti-Nicene Church* (London, 1940).

Frost, R., *Christ and Wholeness* (Cambridge, 1985).

Fulford, K.W.M., "Praxis Makes Perfect: Illness as a Bridge Between Biological Concepts of Disease and Social Conceptions of Health", in: *Theoretical Medicine*, 14/4 (1993), 305–320.

Gadamer, H.-G., *Schmerz: Einschätzungen aus medizinischer, philosophischer und therapeutischer Sicht* (Heidelberg, 2003).

Gadamer, H.-G., *Über die Verborgenheit der Gesundheit* (Frankfurt, 2003).

Galen, *Mixtures,* trans. P.N. Singer, in: Selected works (Oxford, 1997), 202–289.

Galen, *The Affections and Errors of the Soul*, trans. P.N. Singer, in: Selected works (Oxford, 1997), 100–149.

Galen, *The Art of Medicine*, trans. P.N. Singer, in: Selected works (Oxford, 1997), 345–396.

Galen, *The Best Constitution of Our Bodies*, trans. P.N. Singer, in: Selected works (Oxford, 1997), 290–295.

Galen, *The Best Doctor is Also a Philosopher*, trans. P.N. Singer, in: Selected works (Oxford, 1997), 30–34.

Galen, *The Order of My Own Books*, trans. P.N. Singer, in: Selected works (Oxford, 1997), 23–29.

Galen, *The Pulse for Beginners,* trans. P.N. Singer, in: Selected works (Oxford, 1997), 325–344.

Galen, *The Soul's Dependence on the Body*, trans. P.N. Singer, in: Selected works (Oxford, 1997), 150–176.

Galen, *To Thrasyboulos: Is Healthiness a Part of Medicine or Gymnastics?* trans. P.N. Singer, in: Selected works (Oxford, 1997), 53–99.

Galen, *On the Therapeutic Method: Books I and II*, trans. R.J. Hankinson (Oxford 1991).

Geerlings, W., *Theologen der christlichen Antike* (Darmstadt, 2002).

Gillett, C./Loewer, B. (eds.), *Physicalism and Its Discontents* (Cambridge, 2001).

Gilson, E., *The Christian philosophy of St. Augustine* (London, 1961).

Gregory of Nazianzus, *On his Brother, St. Caesarius*, trans. L.P. McCauley, in: Fathers of the Church, 22 (Washington, 1953).

Gregory of Nazianzus, *On St. Basil the Great, Bishop of Caesarea*, trans. L.P. McCauley, in: Fathers of the Church, 22 (Washington, 1953).

Gregory of Nyssa, *On Virginity*, trans. V. Woods Callahan, in: Fathers of the Church, 58 (Washington, 1967).

Gregory of Nyssa, *On the Soul and the Resurrection*, trans. V. Woods Callahan, in: Fathers of the Church, 58 (Washington, 1967).

Guttmacher, S., "Whole in Body, Mind and Spirit: Holistic Health and the Limits of Medicine", in: *The Hastings Center Report* (1979), 15–21.

Guyton, A.C./Hall, J.E., *Textbook of Medical Physiology* (Philadelphia, [11]2006).

Habermas, J., *The Future of Human Nature*, trans W. Rehg/M. Pensky/H. Beister (Cambridge/Malden, 2003).

Hamman, A.-G., *L'homme, image de dieu. Essay d'une anthropologie chrétienne dans l'eglise des cinq premiers siècles* (Paris, 1987).

Harakas, S., *Towards Transfigured Life: The Theoria of Eastern Orthodox Ethics* (Minneapolis 1983).

Harakas, S., *Wholeness of Faith and Life: Orthodox Christian Ethics. Part One: Patristic Ethics* (Brookline, 1999).

Harakas, S., *Health and Medicine in the Eastern Orthodox Tradition* (Crossroads/New York, 2000).

Harig, G./Kolesch, J., "Arzt, Kranker, und Krankenpflege in der griechisch-römischen Antike und im byzantinischen Mittelalter", in: *Helikon* 13/14 (1973/74), 256–292.

Harig, G., "Zum Problem 'Krankenhaus' in der Antike", in: *Klio* 53 (1971), 179–195.

Harnack, A., "Medicinisches aus Ältester Kirchengeschichte", in: *Texte und Untersuchungen zur Geschichte der altchristlichen Literatur*, 8 (1892), 37–152.

Harrison, C., *Augustine. Christian Truth and Fractured Humanity* (Oxford, 2000).

Hauerwas, S./Burrell, D., "From System to Story: An Alternative Pattern for Rationality in Ethics", in: *The Roots of Ethics. Science, Religion and Values*, ed. Engelhardt/Callahan (New York, 1981), 75–105.

Hauerwas, S., "Salvation and Health: Why Medicine Needs the Church", in: *Philosophy and Medicine*, 20 (1985), 205–224.

Hauerwas, S., *Naming the Silences. God, Medicine, and the Problem of Suffering* (Edinburgh, 1993).

Hauschild, W.-D., *Gottes Geist und der Mensch. Studien zur frühchristlichen Pneumatologie*, in: Beiträge zur evangelischen Theologie, 63 (Munich, 1972).

Heijke, J., *St. Augustine's Comments on "Imago Dei" - An Anthology from all his Works Exclusive of the De Trinities* (1960).

Hesslow, G., "Do We need a Concept of Disease?" in: *Theoretical Medicine*, 14/1 (1993), 1–14.

Hippocrates, *Airs, Waters, Places*, trans. J. Chadwick/W.N. Mann, in: Hippocratic Writings, ed. G.E.R. Lloyd (London, 1983), 148–169.

Hippocrates, *The Nature of Man*, trans. J. Chadwick/W.N. Mann, in: Hippocratic Writings, ed. G.E.R. Lloyd (London, 1983), 260–271.

Hippocrates, *The Oath*, trans. J. Chadwick/W.N. Mann, in: Hippocratic Writings, ed. G.E.R. Lloyd (London, 1983), 67–68.

Hippocrates, *The Science of Medicine*, trans. J. Chadwick/W.N. Mann, in: Hippocratic Writings, ed. G.E.R. Lloyd (London, 1983), 139–147.

Hippocrates *Tradition in Medicine*, trans. J. Chadwick/W.N. Mann, in: Hippocratic Writings, ed. G.E.R. Lloyd (London, 1983), 70–86.

Hogan, R.M./LeVoir, J.M., *Covenant of Love. Pope John Paul II on Sexuality, Marriage, and Family in the Modern World* (San Francisco, 1992).

Holland, S./Lebacqz, K./Sloth, L., The *Human Embryonic Stem Cell Debate: Science, Ethics, and Public Policy* (Cambridge, MA 2001).

Holman, S.R., *The Hungry are Dying* (Oxford, 2001).

Holmes, A., *A Life Pleasing to God: The Spirituality of the Rules of St Basil* (London, 2000).

Hombert, P.M., *Nouvelles Recherches de Chronologies*, in: Collection des Etudes Augustinian's (2000).

House of Commons: Science & Technology Committee, *Human Reproductive Technologies and the Law. Fifth report of session 2004-05* (London, 2005).

House of Lords, *Stem Cell Research: Report from the Select Committee* (London, 2002).

Human Fertilisation and Embryology Act 1990 c. 37 (London, 1990), www.hmso.gov.uk/acts/-acts1990/Ukpga_19900037_en_1.htm.

Human Fertilisation and Embryology Authority/Human Genetics Advisory Commission, *Cloning Issues in Reproduction, Science and Medicine: A Consultation Document* (London, 1998).

Illich, I., *Limits to Medicine. Medical Nemesis: The Expropriation of Health* (London/New York, 1976).

Illich, I., "The Institutional Construction of a New Fetish: Human Life", in: *In the Mirror of the Past: Lectures and Addresses 1978–1990*, ed. I. Illich (London/New York, 1992), 218–232.

Illich, I., "Twelve Years after Medical Nemesis: a Plea for Body History", in: *In the Mirror of the Past: Lectures and Addresses 1978–1990*, ed. I. Illich (London/New York, 1992), 211–217.

Irenaeus, *Against Heresies*, trans. J. Keble (Oxford, 1872).

Jackson, R., *Doctors and Diseases in the Roman Empire* (London, 1988).

Jaspers, K., *Plato and Augustine* (New York/London, 1962).

Jiang, Y. et al., "Pluripotency of Mesenchymal Stem Cells Derived from Adult Marrow", in: *Nature*, 418 (2002), 41–49.

Joest, W., *Dogmatik* (Göttingen, 1996).

John Paul II, *On the Christian Meaning of Human Suffering*, English trans. (Boston, 1984).

John Paul II, *Evangelium Vitae. The Value and Inviolability of Human Life,* English trans. (London, 1995).

John Paul II, *The Theology of the Body. Human Love in the Divine Plan,* English trans. (Boston, 1997).

John Paul II, *Contemplate the Face of Christ in the Sick*, English trans. (London, 2000).

Jones, C./Porter, R., *Reassessing Foucault: Power, Medicine, the Body.* (London/New York, 1994).

Junkers-Kenny, M., "Der moralische Status des Embryo in Kontext der Reproduktionsmedizin", in: *Ethik in der Humangenetik*, ed. Mieth/Düwell (Tübingen/Basel, 1998), 302–323.

Kahn, A., "Therapeutic Cloning and the Status of the Embryo", in: *Ethical eye-Cloning*, 2 (2002), 103–118.

Kappa, U./Mertelsmann, R., "Plasticity of Stem Cells", in: *Stem Cells from Cord Blood, in uteri Stem Cell Development and Transplantation-Inclusive Gene Therapy*, ed. W. Holzgreve/M. Less(Heidelberg, 2001), 1–18.

Kass, L.R., "Regarding the End of Medicine and the Pursuit of Health", in: *The Public Interest*, 40 (1975), 11–42.

Kass, L.R./Wilson, J.Q., *The Ethics of Human Cloning* (Washington, 1998).

Kee, H.C., *Medicine, Miracle and Magic in New Testament Times* (Cambridge, 1986).

Keller, S.R., "A Sociocultural Concept of Health", in: *The Journal of Medicine and Philosophy*, 1/3 (1976), 222–228.

Keenan, M.E., *The life and times of St. Augustine as revealed in his letters* (Washington, 1935).

Keenan, M.E., "St. Gregory of Nazianzus and early Byzantine Medicine", in: *Bulletin of the History of Medicine*, 9 (1941), 8–30.

Keenan, M.E., "St. Gregory of Nyssa and the Medical Profession", in: *Bulletin of the History of Medicine*, 15 (1944), 150–161.

Kelsey, M.T., *Healing and Christianity in Ancient Thought and Modern Times* (London, 1973).

Khushf, G., "Expanding the Horizon of Reflection on Health and Disease", in: *Journal of Medicine and Philosophy*, 20/5 (1995), 461–473.

Kierkegaard, S., *Fear and Trembling*, trans. A. Haunay (London 1985).

Knuuttila, S., "Time and Creation in Augustine", in: *The Cambridge Companion to Augustine*, ed. E. Stump/N. Kretzmann (Cambridge, 2001), 103–115.

Krug, A., *Heilkunst und Heilkult. Medizin in der Antike* (München, 1984).

Kudlien, F., "Galen's Religious Belief", in: *Galen. Problems and Prospects*, ed. V. Nutton (London, 1981), 117–130.

Lander, G.B., "St. Augustine's Conception of the Reformation of Man to the Image of God", in: *Augustinus Magister: Congrès International Augustinian, Paris, 21–24 September 1954*, 2 (1954), 867–878.

Lamberigts, M., "Julian of Eclanum", in: *Augustine Through the Ages: An Encyclopaedia*, ed. A.D. Fitzgerald (Grand Rapids/Cambridge, 1999), 478–479.

Lanzerath, D./Honnefelder, L., "Krankheitsbegriff und ärztliche Anwendung der Humangenetik", in: *Ethik in der Humangenetik*, ed. Mieth, D./Düwell, M. (Tübingen/Basel, 1998), 51–77.

Lanzerath, D., *Krankheit und ärztliches Handeln. Zur Funktion des Krankheitsbegriffs in der medizinischen Ethik* (Freiburg/München, 2000).

Lavère, G.J., "Camus' Plague and Saint Augustine's *Civitas Terrenae*", in: *Proceedings of the PMR Conference*, 10 (1985), 87–98.

Leahy, D.J., *St. Augustine on Eternal Life* (London, 1939).

Lennox, J.G., "Health as an Objective Value", in: *Journal of Medicine and Philosophy*, 20/5 (1995), 499–511.

Lieb, I.C., "The Image of Man in Medicine", in: *The Journal of Medicine and Philosophy*, 1/2 (1976), 162–176.

Lindberg, D., "Science and the Early Church", in: *God and Nature. Historical Essays on the Encounter Between Christianity and Science,* ed. D. Lindberg/R.L. Numbers (London, 1986), 19–48.

Lloyd, G.E.R., *Methods and Problems in Greek Science* (Cambridge, 1991).

Lupton, D., *Medicine as Culture: Illness, Disease and the Body in Western Societies* (London, 1994).

MacIntyre, A./Gorovitz, S., "Towards a Theory of Medical Fallibility", in: *The Journal of Medicine and Philosophy*, 1/1 (1976), 51–71.

MacIntyre, A., "Theology, Ethics, and the Ethics of Medicine and Health Care: Comments on Papers by Novak, Mow, Roach, Cahilll, and Hartt", in: *The Journal of Medicine and Philosophy*, 4/4 (1979), 435–443.

MacIntyre, A., "Can Medicine Dispense with a Theological Perspective on Human Nature?", in: *The Roots of Ethics: Science, Religion and Values*, ed. D. Callahan/H.T. Engelhardt (New York/London 1981), 119–137.

MacIntyre, A., *After Virtue. A Study in Moral Theory* (London, 1985).

Macqueen, D.J., "Contemptus Dei: St. Augustine on the Disorder of Pride in Society, and Its Remedies", in: *Recherches Augustinian's*, 9 (1973), 223–242.

Martens, G., "Augustine's Image of Man", in: *Images of Man in Ancient and Medieval Thought*, ed. F. Bossier (Leuven, 1976), 127–146.

Makoth, M., "Galen als Seelenheiler", in: *Galen und das hellenistische Erbe. Verhandlungen des IV. Internationalen Galen Symposium 1989*, ed. Kollesch, J./Nickel, R. (Stuttgart, 1993), 145–156.

Margolis, J., "The Concept of Disease", in: *The Journal of Medicine and Philosophy*, 1/3 (1976), 238–268.

Markus, R.A., "'Imago' and 'Similitudo' in Augustine", in: *Revue des Études Augustinian's*, 10/2–3 (1964), 125–143.

Markus, R.A., *Speculum. History and Society in the Theology of St Augustine* (Cambridge, 1970).

Markus, R.A., *Sacred and Secular* (Vermont, 1994).

Marty, M.E., *Health and Medicine in the Lutheran Tradition* (Crossroads/New York, 1998).

Mascall, E.L., *The Triune God. An Ecumenical Study* (Worthing, 1986).

Mathewes, C.T., *Evil and the Augustinian Tradition* (Cambridge, 2001).

Matthews, G.B., "The Inner Man", in: *Augustine: A Collection of Critical Essays*, ed. R.A. Markus (New York, 1972), 176–190.

Marrow, H.I., *The Resurrection and Saint Augustine's Theology of Human Values* (Villanova, 1966).

McCormick, R., "Who or What is the Pre-embryo?", in: *Kennedy Institute of Ethics Journal*, 1/1 (1991), 1–15.

McGee, G./Kaplan, A., "The Ethics and Politics of Small Sacrifices in Stem cell Research", in: *Kennedy Institute of Ethics Journal*, 9/2 (1999), 151–158.

Meilaender, G., "*Terra es animata*: On Having a Life", in: *Hastings Center Report*, 23/4 (1993), 23–32.

Meilaender, G., "Second Thoughts about Body Parts", in: *First Things*, 62 (1996), 32–37.

Meilaender, G., "Begetting and Cloning", in: *First Things*, 74 (1997), 41–43.

Meilaender, G., *Body, Soul, and Bioethics* (Notre Dame/London, 1998).

Meilaender, G., "The Point of a Ban: Or, How to Think about Stem Cell Research", in: *Hastings Center Report*, 31/1 (2001), 9–16.

Meilaender, G., "Designing our Descendants", in: *First Things*, 109 (2001), 25–28.

Meilaender, G., "Between Beasts and God", in: *First Things*, 119 (2002), 23–29.

Meilaender, G., "In Search of Wisdom: Bioethics and the Character of Human Life". Paper discussed at The President's Council on Bioethics January 2002 meeting. http://www.bioethics.gov/meilaenderpaper.html

Menn, S., *Descartes and Augustine* (Cambridge, 1998).

Meyer, M.J./Nelson, L.J., "Respecting what we Destroy: Reflections on Human Embryo Research", in: *Hastings Center Report*, 31/1 (2001), 16–23.

Mieth, D., "Ethics, Morality and Religion", in: *Ethical eye-Cloning*, 1 (2002), 119–140.

Miles, M.R., *Plotinus on Body and Beauty: Society, Philosophy, and Religion in Third Century Rome* (Oxford, 1999).

Mill, J.S., *Utilitarianism* (London, 1967).

Miller, T.S., *The Birth of the Hospital in the Byzantine Empire* (London/Baltimore, 1985).

Müller, A.M. et al., "Origin and Developmental Plasticity of Hematopoietic Stem Cells", in: *Stem Cells from Cord Blood, in Uteri Stem Cell Development and Transplantation - Inclusive Gene Therapy*, ed. W. Holzgreve/M. Less (Heidelberg, 2001), 29–46.

Moser, P.K./Trout, J.D. (eds.), *Contemporary Materialism: A Reader* (London/New York, 1995).

Moraux, P., "Galien comme philosophe: la philosophie de la nature", in: *Galen. Problems and Prospects*, ed. V. Nutton (London, 1981), 87–116.

Moraux, P., "Galien et Aristotle", in: *Images of Man in Ancient and Medieval Thought*, ed. F. Bossier (Leuven, 1976), 175–198.

Moravcsik, J., "Ancient and Modern Conceptions of Health and Medicine", in: *The Journal of Medicine and Philosophy*, 1/4 (1976), 337–348.

Mordacci, R., "Health as an Analogical Concept", in: *The Journal of Medicine and Philosophy*, 20/5 (1995), 475–497.

Nagel, T., "What is it Like to be a Bat?", in: *The Philosophical Review*, 83/4 (1974), 435–450.

National Bioethics Advisory Commission, *Ethical Issues in Human Stem Cell Research: Report and Recommendations of the National Bioethics Advisory Commission* (Rockville, Maryland, 1999).

National Bioethics Advisory Commission, *Cloning Human Beings: Report and Recommendations of the National Bioethics Advisory Commission* (Rockville, Maryland, 1997).

National Institutes of Health, *Stem Cells: A Primer* (Washington, 2002).

National Institutes of Health, *Scientific Progress and Future Research Directions* (Washington, 2001).

Nationaler Ethikrat, *Zum Import menschlicher embryonaler Stammzellen. Stellungnahme* (Berlin, 2002).

Nietzsche, F., *Beyond Good and Evil* (London, 1973).

Nordenfelt, L., "On the Relevance and Importance of the Notion of Disease", in: *Theoretical Medicine*, 14/1 (1993), 15–26.

Nordenfelt, L., "Concepts of Health and their Consequences for Health Care", in: *Theoretical Medicine*, 14/4 (1993), 277–285.

Nordenfelt, L., *On the Notion of Health. An Action-Theoretic Approach* (Dordrecht, 1994).

Nuffield Council on Bioethics, *Stem Cell Therapy: The Ethical Issues. A Discussion Paper* (London, 2000).

Nüsslein-Vollhardt, C., *Von Genen und Embryonen* (Stuttgart, 2004).

Nutton, V., "The Chronology of Galen's Early Career", in: *The Classical Quarterly*, XXIII/1 (1973), 158–171.

Nutton, V., "Murders and Miracles: Lay Attitudes to Medicine in Classical Antiquity, in: *Patients and Perceptions: Lay Perceptions of Medicine in Pre-Industrial Society*, ed. R. Porter (Cambridge, 1985), 23–54.

Nutton, V., "Style and Context in the *Method of Healing*", in: *Galen's Method of Healing. Proceedings of the 1982 Galen Symposium*, ed. F. Kudlien/R.J. Durling (Leiden/New York, 1991), 1–25.

O'Connell, R.J., *The Origin of the Soul in St. Augustine's Later Works* (New York, 1987).

O'Donovan, O., *Begotten or Made?* (Oxford, 1984).

O'Donovan, O., "Again: Who Is a Person?", in: *Abortion and the Sanctity of Human Life*, ed. J.H. Channer (Exeter, 1985), 125–137.

O'Donovan, O., *Resurrection and Moral Order* (Leicester, 1996).

O'Donovan, O., "Keeping Body and Soul Together", in: *Philosophy and Medicine*, 77 (2002), 35–54.

O'Rahilly, R./Müller, F., *Human Embryology and Teratology* (New York, 2001).

Origen, *Contra Celsum*, trans. H. Chadwick (Cambridge, 1953).

Outka, G., "The Ethics of Stem Cell Research"-Paper discussed at the President's Council on Bioethics April 2002 meeting. http://www.bioethics.gov/outka.html.

Parry, S., "The Politics of Cloning: Mapping the Rhetorical Convergence of Embryos and Stem Cells in Parliamentary Debates", in: *New Genetics and Society*, 22/2 (2003), 177–200.

Pegs, A.C., "The Mind of St. Augustine", in: *Medieval Studies*, 6 (1944), 23–48.

Pellegrino, E., "Toward a Reconstruction of Medical Morality: The Primacy of the Act of Profession and the Fact of Illness", in: *The Journal of Medicine and Philosophy*, 4/1 (1979), 32–56.

Pellegrino, E./Thomasma, D., *A Philosophical Basis of Medical Practice: Toward a Philosophy and Ethic of the Healing Profession* (New York/Oxford, 1981).

Pelikan, J., *The Christian Tradition: A History of the Development of Doctrine* (Chicago, 1974).

Pelikan, J., *Christianity and Classical Culture: The Metamorphosis of Natural Theology in the Christian Encounter with Hellenism* (New Haven/London, 1993).

Perkins, J., *The Suffering Self: Pain and Narrative Representation in the Early Christian Era* (London/New York, 1995).

Petersson, B., "Health, Doctors and the Good Life: a Footnote to Plato", in: *Dimensions of Health and Health Promotion*, ed. L. Nordenfelt (Amsterdam/New York, 2003), 3–22.

Plato, *Republic*, trans. R. Waterfield (Oxford, 1993).

Plato, *Symposium*, trans. R. Waterfield (Oxford, 1994).

Plato, *Timaeus*, trans. H.D.P. Lee (London, 1965).

Porter, R., *The Greatest Benefit to Mankind: A Medical History of Humanity from Antiquity to Present* (London, 1995).

Porter, R., "Hospitals and Surgery", in: *The Cambridge Illustrated History of Medicine*, ed. R. Porter (Cambridge, 1996), 202–245.

Porter, R., *Religion, Healing, and Suffering* (London/New York, 1999).

Quasten, J., *Patrology*, Vol. I-IV (Westminster/Maryland, 1994[7])

Ramsey, P., *Fabricated Man: The Ethics of Genetic Control* (New Haven/London, 1970).

Ramsey, P., *The Ethics of Fetal Research* (London/New Haven, 1975).

Rather, J. et al., "Lineage Specific Differentiation of Pluripotent Cells *In Vitro*: A Role for Extraembryonic Cell Types", in: *Reproduction, Fertility and Development*, 13/1 (2001), 15–22.

Rawls, J., "Two Concepts of Rules", in: *The Philosophical Review*, 6 (1955), 3–32.

Rundle-Short, A., *The Bible and Modern Medicine: A Survey of Health and Healing in the Old and New Testament* (London, 1953).

Ricoeur, P., *The Symbolism of Evil*, trans. E. Buchanan (Boston, 1967).

Rideout III, W.M. et al., "Correction of a Genetic Defect by Nuclear Transplantation and Combined Cell and Gene Therapy", in: *Cell*, 109/1 (2002), 17–27.

Riede, U.-N./Schaefer, H.-E., *Allgemeine und spezielle Pathologie* (Stuttgart/New York, 1995).

Rigby, P., *Original Sin in Augustine's Confessions* (Ottawa, 1987).

Risse, G.B., *Mending Bodies, Saving Souls: A History of Hospitals* (London/New York, 1999).

Risse, G.B., "Health and Disease: History of the Concepts", in: *Encyclopaedia of Bioethics*, ed. W.T. Reich, (1995), 579–585.

Rist, J.M., *Human Value: A Study in Ancient Philosophical Ethics* (Leiden, 1982).

Rist, J.M., *Augustine: Ancient Thought Baptized* (Cambridge, 1994).

Rist, J.M., *Man, Soul, and Body: Essays in Ancient Thought from Plato to Dionysios* (Leiden, 1996).

Robertson, J.A., "Ethics and Policy in Embryonic Stem Cell Research", in: *Kennedy Institute of Ethics Journal*, 9/2 (1999), 109–136.

Rothschuh, K.E. (ed.), *Was ist Krankheit? Erscheinung, Erklärung, Sinndeutung* (Darmstadt, 1995).

Royal Society, *Stem Cell Research and Therapeutic Cloning: An Update* (London, 2000).

Royal Society, *Therapeutic Cloning. A Submission by the Royal Society to the Chief Medical Officer's Expert Group* (London, 2000).

Royal Society, *Stem Cell Research: Second Update* (London, 2001).

Ruokanen, M., *Theology of Social Life in Augustine's De civitate Dei*, in: Forschungen zur Kirchen-und Dogmengeschichte, 53 (1993).

Sade, R., "A Theory of Health and Disease: the Objectivist-Subjectivist Dichotomy", in: *The Journal of Medicine and Philosophy*, 20/5 (1995), 512–525.

Schäfer, D./Frewer, A./Schockenhoff, E./Wetzstein, V. (eds.), *Gesundheitskonzepte im Wandel. Geschichte, Ethik und Gesellschaft,* in: Geschichte und Philosophie der Medizin, Vol. 6 (Stuttgart, 2008).

Scheffczyk, L., *Der Mensch als Bild Gottes* (Darmstadt, 1969).

Schmidt, U./Frewer, A. (eds.), *History and Theory of Human Experimentation. The Declaration of Helsinki and Modern Medical Ethics*, in: Geschichte und Philosophie der Medizin, Vol. 2 (Stuttgart, 2007).

Schuchardt, E. et al., *Was macht den Menschen krank* (Basel/Berlin/Boston, 1991).

Schipperges, H./Seidler, E./Unschuld, P.U., *Krankheit, Heilkunst, Heilung* (Freiburg/Munich, 1978).

Schweizer, E., "σαρξ"/ "σωμα", in: *Theologisches Wörterbuch zum Neuen Testament*, ed. G. Friedrich, VII (Stuttgart, 1964), 123–151/1054–1091.

Seidl, H., "Seele V: Kirchen-und philosophiegeschichtlich", in: *Theologische Realenzyklopädie*, ed. G. Müller, XXX (Berlin, 1999), 748–759.

Shamblott, M.J. et al., "Derivation of Pluripotent Stem Cells from Cultured Human Primordial Germ Cells", in: *Proceedings of the National Academy of Sciences*, 95 (1998), 13726–13731.

Siegel, R.E., *Galen's System of Physiology and Medicine: An Analysis of his Doctrines and Observations on Blood Flow, Respiration, Humors and Internal Diseases* (Basel/Munich, 1968).

Siegel, R.E., *Galen on Sense Perception: His Doctrines, Observations, Experiments on Vision, Hearing, Smell, Taste, Touch and Pain and Their Historical Sources* (Basel/Munich, 1970).

Siegel, R.E., *Galen on Psychology, Psychopathology, and Function and Diseases of the Nervous System: An Analysis of his Doctrines, Observations and Experiments* (Basel/Munich, 1973).

Siegler, M., "The Doctor-Patient Encounter and Its Relationship to Theories of Health and Disease", in: *Concepts of Health and Disease. Interdisciplinary Perspectives*, ed. A.L. Caplan/H.T. Engelhardt/J.J. McCartney (Reading/Masachusetts, 1981), 627–644.

Singer, P.N., *Galen on the Soul: Philosophy and Medicine in the Second Century A.D.* PhD-thesis. (Cambridge, 1992).

Smart, J.J.C., "Extreme and Restricted Utilitarianism", in: *Theories of Ethics*, ed. P. Foot, (Oxford, 1967).

Smith, W.D., *The Hippocratic Tradition* (London, 1979).

Sonntag, S., *Illness as Metaphor* (New York, 1977).

Song, R., "To Be Willing to Kill What for All One Knows Is A Person Is to Be Willing to Kill a Person", in: *God and the Embryo: Religious Voices on Stem Cells and Cloning*, ed. B. Waters/R.Cole-Turner (Washington, 2003), 98–107.

Stiker, H.J., *A History of Disability*, trans. W. Sayers (Ann Arbor, 1999).

Sullivan, J.E., *The Image of God: The Doctrine of St. Augustine and Its Influence.* (Dubuque, 1963).

Tatian, *Oratio ad Graecos and Fragments*, trans. M. Whittaker, in: Oxford Early Christian Texts (Oxford, 1982).

Temkin, O., "Health and Disease", in: *Dictionary of the History of Ideas*, ed. P. Wiener, III (1973), 395–407.

Temkin, O., *Hippocrates in a World of Pagans and Christians* (Baltimore, 1991).

Tertullian, *Homily on Baptism*, trans. E. Evans (London, 1964).

Tertullian, *Tertullian's Treatise on the Resurrection*, trans. E. Evans (London, 1960).

Tertullian, *The Chaplet*, trans. E. A. Quain, in: The Fathers of the Church, 40 (Washington, 1959).

Tertullian, *Flight in Time of Persecution*, trans. E. A. Quain, in: The Fathers of the Church, 40 (Washington, 1959).

Tertullian, *Apology*, trans. Sr. E. J. Daily, in: The Fathers of the Church, 10 (Washington, 1950).

Tertullian, *The Antidote to the Scorpion's Bite*, trans. A. Roberts/J. Donaldson, in: Ante-Nicene Christian Library, 11 (Edinburgh, 1869).

Teselle, E., *Augustine the Theologian* (London, 1970).

Teske, R., "Augustine's Theory of the Soul", in: *The Cambridge Companion to Augustine*, ed. E. Stump/N. Kretzmann, (Cambridge, 2001), 116–123.

The Nuremberg Code, 1947, bmj.bmjjournals.com/cgi/content/full/313/7070/1448.

The President's Council on Bioethics, Transcripts from The President's Council on Bioethics meetings (2002-2004), http://www.bioethics.gov/transcripts.

The President's Council on Bioethics, *Human Cloning and Human Dignity: an Ethical Inquiry* (Washington, 2002).

The President's Council on Bioethics, *Beyond Therapy: Biotechnology and the Pursuit of Happiness: a Report by The President's Council on Bioethics* (Washington, 2003).

The President's Council on Bioethics, *Monitoring Stem Cell Research: a Report of The President's Council on Bioethics* (Washington, 2004).

The Wellcome Trust, *Public Perceptions on Human Cloning* (London, 1998).

Thomas Aquinas, *Basic Writings*, ed. A.C. Pegis, I & II (Indianapolis/Cambridge, 1997).

Thomson, J.A. et al., "Embryonic Stem Cell Lines Derived from Human Blastocysts", in: *Science*, 282 (1998), 1145–1147.

Tillich, P., "The Relation of Religion and Health: Historical Considerations and Theoretical Questions", in: *Review of Religion,* 10 (1946), 348–384.

Timothy, H.B., *Early Christian Apologists and Greek Philosophy* (Assen, 1973).

Toombs, S.K., *The Meaning of Illness. A Phenomenological Account of the Different Perspectives of Physician and Patient*, in: Philosophy and Medicine, 42 (1992).

Toulmin, S., "Concepts of Function and Mechanism in Medicine and Medical Science (Hommage à Claude Bernard)", in: *Philosophy and Medicine*, 1 (1975), 51–66.

Toulmin, S., "On the Nature of the Physician's Understanding", in: *The Journal of Medicine and Philosophy*, 1/1 (1976), 32–50.

Trounson, A.O., "Nuclear Transfer in Human Medicine and Animal Breeding", in: *Reproduction, Fertility and Development*, 13/1 (2001), 31–40.

UK Stem Cell Initiative, *Report and Recommendations* (London 2005).

UNESCO, *Declaration on the Human Genome and Human Rights*, http://www. portal.unesco.org

Walzer, R., *Galen on Jews and Christians* (Oxford, 1949).

Warnock, M., *A Question of Life: The Warnock Report on Human Fertilisation and Embryology with Two New Chapters* (London, 1985).

Weaver, R. H., "Prayer", in: *Augustine Through the Ages: an Encyclopedia*, ed. A.D. Fitzgerald (Grand Rapids/Cambridge, 1999), 670–675.

Weber, D., "Augustinus, *De Genesi Contra Manichaeos*. Zu Augustins Darstellung und Widerlegung der Manichäischen Kritik am biblischen Schöpfungbericht", in: *Augustine and Manichaeism in the Latin West. Proceedings of the Fribourg-Utrecht International Symposium of the IAMS*, ed. van Oort/Wermelinger/Wurst (Leiden/Boston, 2001), 298–306.

Wetzel, J., *Augustine and the Limits of Virtue* (Cambridge, 1992).

Wetzel, J., "Predestination, Pelagianism, and Foreknowledge", in: *The Cambridge Companion to Augustine*, ed. Stump/Kretzmann (Cambridge, 2001), 49–58.

Wiesing, U., "Gene, Krankheit, und Moral", in: *Ethik in der Humangenetik*, ed. Mieth/Düwell (Tübingen/Basel, 1998), 78–87.

Williams, B., *Morality: An Introduction to Ethics* (Cambridge, 1972).

Williams, B./Smart, J.J.C., *Utilitarianism – For and Against* (Cambridge, 1973).

Williams, B., *Utilitarianism and Beyond* (Cambridge, 1982).

Williams, B., *Plato: The Invention of Philosophy* (London, 1998).

Wunder, E., "Chances and Limits of Cord Blood Transplantation", in: *Stem Cells from Cord Blood, In Utero Stem Cell Development and Transplantation-Inclusive Gene Therapy*, ed. Holzgreve/Lessl (Heidelberg, 2001), 71–84.

Zaner, R.M., "Context and Reflexivity: The Genealogy of Self", in: *Evaluation and Explanation in the Biomedical Sciences,* ed. Engelhardt, T./Spicker, E. (Dordrecht 1975), 153–174.

INDEX

GESCHICHTE UND PHILOSOPHIE DER MEDIZIN /
HISTORY AND PHILOSOPHY OF MEDICINE

Herausgegeben von Andreas Frewer.

Franz Steiner Verlag   ISSN 1860–6199